T0078074

How to Overcome INSOMNIA All by Yourself

*A Healthy Sense of Self Guide
to Getting a Good Night's Sleep*

ANTOINETTA VOGELS

BALBOA.PRESS
A DIVISION OF HAY HOUSE

Balboa Press books may be ordered through booksellers or by contacting:

Balboa Press
A Division of Hay House
1663 Liberty Drive
Bloomington, IN 47403
www.balboapress.com
844-682-1282

Because of the dynamic nature of the Internet, any web addresses or links contained in this book may have changed since publication and may no longer be valid. The views expressed in this work are solely those of the author and do not necessarily reflect the views of the publisher, and the publisher hereby disclaims any responsibility for them.

The author of this book does not dispense medical advice or prescribe the use of any technique as a form of treatment for physical, emotional, or medical problems without the advice of a physician, either directly or indirectly. The intent of the author is only to offer information of a general nature to help you in your quest for emotional and spiritual well-being. In the event you use any of the information in this book for yourself, which is your constitutional right, the author and the publisher assume no responsibility for your actions.

Print information available on the last page.

ISBN: 978-1-9822-4448-4 (sc)
ISBN: 978-1-9822-4450-7 (hc)
ISBN: 978-1-9822-4449-1 (e)

Library of Congress Control Number: 2020904477

Balboa Press rev. date: 02/22/2022

CONTENTS

I dedicate this book to:

All people
who suffer from insomnia.

All those who are unable to replenish their
energy and vitality and therefore find it
impossible to fully flourish in their lives.

All the parents
who do their best to raise their children
while being unable to rest their minds and bodies at night.

All the children
whose parents are too tired and
preoccupied to give their kids
the attention they deserve because they
didn't get a good night's sleep.

All the weary travelers on the road
who are a potential danger to themselves and others
because they aren't as alert in traffic as
they would be if they could sleep.

All the employees
whose decisions or leadership is questioned
because of their chronic fatigue.

All the laborers
who go to work feeling so tired
that they become more prone to accidents.

All the retirees
who find it hard to stay active or take
pleasure in their golden years
because they can't sleep or they wake up too early.

All my fellow men and women
who struggle to get the sleep they
need and are deeply troubled
by the consequences of their
unwanted nightly wakefulness.

AUTHOR'S NOTE

When I first began looking into the concept of the sense of self, there was no information available, and I had to connect the dots on my own. Thankfully, quite a lot of research has been done since the early nineties, and now there's a wealth of academic knowledge that confirms my conclusions.

My most notable research discovery was also my most recent one: *The Body Keeps the Score* by Bessel van der Kolk, MD. His decades of research in the fields of psychology and neuroscience gave me a fantastic sense of validation in my own personal findings and deeper insight into why those of us with childhood trauma think, feel, behave, and react to things the way we do.[1]

Unfortunately, due to the timing of this discovery, I wasn't able to include references to his work in this book. However, I'm deeply grateful to Dr. van der Kolk for the insight he's brought to this topic. I hope you'll take the time to read his work to deepen your knowledge of the inner workings of your own mind and emotions by learning more about how adverse childhood experiences and PTSD affect the brain and how it adapts to trauma.

Knowledge is power, and with all the information that's so easily available now, you don't have to be an expert in psychology to understand what's going on within yourself. Although my voice doesn't have the label of "doctor" in front of it, I still managed to find the truth through determination and hard work. You can too. While this book reflects my personal background of not receiving adequate mental and emotional care in childhood, the Sense of Self (SoS) Method can be a valuable resource for anyone suffering from the consequences of a painful childhood.

> "Not being seen, not being known, and having nowhere to turn to feel safe is devastating at any age, but it is particularly destructive for young children, who are still trying to find their place in the world."
> –Bessel van der Kolk, *The Body Keeps the Score*

How to Cure Your Insomnia with the Sense of Self Method

There are a lot of books on the topic of insomnia, but people still can't seem to get a clear understanding of what causes it and how to solve it.

When you seek medical help, doctors usually end up prescribing sleeping pills, but they don't assist you with getting to the root of the issue. Psychologists do their best to help you understand the problem so you can solve it, but what causes a sleeping problem usually lies hidden in the complex constellation of your personal experiences that are stored in your subconscious mind. Thoroughly researching these issues together with a professional requires a lot of time, money, and endurance, which is simply not an option for most of us. That's why, in our day and age, it has become increasingly desirable to take matters into our own hands.

If you're committed to solving the riddle of your insomnia, you've found the right book. Get ready to dive into your past and review the childhood conclusions that are still affecting you today. With the SoS Method, as described in the chapters that follow, you will gradually unlock what keeps you awake at night when you should be soundly asleep, recharging your battery with vital energy.

Living with insomnia can be a lonely experience since no one else really understands what you're going through unless they've experienced it firsthand. It's not just that you can't sleep; insomnia holds you hostage during the day as well. It impacts your thoughts, emotions, and overall quality of life.

As you probably know by now, there's no quick or easy fix for insomnia. It takes real effort and determination to get rid of it for good. But if sleeping problems are disrupting your life, you'd better find the courage to take action.

I lived with insomnia for more than twenty-five years and tried every possible option to get rid of it before I finally figured out how to cure myself. Being able to sleep again gave me my life back. Or let me put it differently: because I reclaimed my life, I was able to sleep again. However, I couldn't stop thinking about all the people who were still living with the agony and isolation of sleepless nights. I felt a strong desire to share my discoveries with other insomniacs and help them recover faster than I did. This is why I created the SoS Method.

I believe that everyone who has a sleeping disorder or who knows someone with insomnia will benefit from reading this book. Working with the SoS Method has a great number of positive side effects. However, this method is especially suitable for solving sleeping problems that are rooted in anxiety that exists on a subconscious level. On the surface, the worries that keep you awake may appear to be about what happened during the day, but you will learn to look at these things from a different angle. A telltale sign that something in your subconscious is responsible for your insomnia is approval-seeking behavior or feeling that your sense of self-worth is tied to living up to certain expectations and conditions.

The ultimate solution lies in being completely yourself. The SoS Method gives you the tools to turn unhealthy patterns of behavior around into self-respecting ones. You will learn to live as your authentic self, which automatically leads to a good night's sleep.

Take the first step. Look within and *heal thy self!*

CHAPTER 1

Not Sleeping—a Curse or a Blessing?

Insomnia can help you find yourself.

If you're reading this, you most likely know firsthand what it feels like when you can't sleep at night. Like me, you've spent hours lying awake, wishing you could sleep, and then forcing yourself to function as well as you possibly can the next day. You too must have experienced those feelings of exhaustion and lethargy. The same resulting frustration, loneliness, stress, and hopelessness, as well as that helpless sense of slowly losing control. Perhaps you've changed since insomnia became a regular part of your life and you've become more sensitive to criticism than you used to be, or you experience the opposite and find yourself feeling emotionally numb.

Insomnia wreaks havoc on your quality of life and it's bad for your overall health, so it's no wonder that sleeping aids are a $29 billion market. People need to sleep. You want to get rid of this problem, but you don't know how. No clear solution has yet been found, and nothing you've tried so far has worked.

As an ex-insomniac, I have written this book to share with you how I managed to get rid of my chronic sleeping problems and hand down the tools that helped me heal myself. It's my deepest wish that you will free yourself from insomnia forevermore.

Let us first agree on how to look at insomnia.

The root cause of insomnia can either be psychological or medical in nature. If there is no medical explanation for your insomnia, understanding the reason you have this problem will allow you to make adjustments to your life and eliminate the issue. I've found that the best way to get started with that is to see insomnia as a type of *self-sabotage*. But note that I don't use this term with the same negative implications that are commonly attributed to it. What I mean to say here is actually the opposite: What if insomnia is, in fact, serving an important natural purpose for you?

This book addresses sleeping problems that are caused by psychological stress due to a *lack of sense of self* and the resulting compensation: dependency on approval. In other words, insomnia can happen when you don't have a strong sense of being your own independent, unique person.

This unfortunate situation usually starts when you're still a child because adverse childhood experiences and developmental trauma[1,2] interfere with the natural development of your sense of self.

Chapter 1

When you don't feel acknowledged as your own unique little person during those early years, an obvious way out is to aim for other people's approval to experience some sense of satisfaction with yourself, or feeling of worthiness. To get approval, you unknowingly force yourself to live up to certain conditions and expectations.[3] This is a core concept of the SoS Method, which I believe is going to help you free yourself from insomnia.

One of the most important discoveries I made is that this state of approval-based feeling of worthiness acts as a kind of artificial, or substitute, sense of self. This is where the concept of self-sabotage comes back in. This self-sabotage can actually be considered nature's way of helping you reject this substitute sense of self so you can find your way back to your *real self*.

I know these viewpoints are quite different from other explanations of what may be causing your sleep disorder. But the role they play in understanding what truly lies behind your inability to sleep will provide the tools you need to tackle it.

While going through my own experience with insomnia, I discovered many truths that weren't obvious to me at first:

- When your *sense of self* is lacking, you often don't feel a real connection with *who you are as your own person*. Instead, you experience temporary feelings of worthiness as a vaguely satisfying substitute for a sense of your real self.
- It's easy to confuse that state of feeling worthy with your own personhood. And having a hard time relating to your real self is what causes this mix-up.

Antoinetta Vogels) 3

- It's necessary to earn other people's approval to experience those temporary feelings of worthiness.
- In the long run, living without a healthy sense of self makes you a slave to approval, which causes you to waste all your energy finding ways to obtain it.
- Your real self is struggling to get free, and, as a result, you instinctually sabotage whatever you were doing to get approval.
- With your sleep being sabotaged, everything you do to gain approval and feel worthy is doomed to fail. This situation forces you to question what's going on with you, which has the potential to help you discover the truth about *why* you do *what* you do.

Because that is the big question! If you want to put an end to your sleeping problems, then ask yourself:

"Why do I do *what* I do?"

"What is my motivation for trying to achieve certain things? Why is it so important for me to fulfill those conditions?" If you can find that out, you are well on your way to freeing yourself from this paralyzing inability to sleep.

I was able to heal myself because I finally came to understand what lay at the root of my insomnia, which ultimately showed me the reasons why I did pretty much everything in my life. It was all about getting acknowledgment. I needed to feel like I mattered, to feel that I was of value instead of a source of problems, instability, and worries. I hope my story releases something inside you that empowers you to reclaim your own life too. I hope that through understanding how things worked for me, you will be motivated to work toward getting to know yourself better. Eventually, it will lead you to going to bed with peace of mind, secure in the knowledge that you will sleep well.

While every person has a vastly different life story, the process of healing is the same. In my case, my path to healing began with the realization that, above all else, I wanted to feel that my parents were happy with me. Instead, I had the strong sense that they found me to be a nuisance.

When I was growing up, it felt as if there was always something wrong with me. I constantly felt pressured because I never seemed to be capable of being on time. I was under the impression my parents thought of me as a self-centered brat who was obsessed with studying to become a good musician. They liked that I was a music student, but the long hours of necessary studying were not really allowed. Hearing me practice at home was too much for them.

The piano was inconveniently placed in the living room, and they really didn't appreciate hearing me play the same piece repeatedly to get it down. They preferred to enjoy their happy hour drinks undisturbed. "Why do you have to be so fanatical about your practicing?" they would ask. "Just be yourself!"

It took me quite some time to figure out that *just be yourself* actually meant *do as we do.*

I never knew an inner feeling of peace, that I was okay. I spent most of my life struggling to acquire that sense and to finally enjoy a good night's sleep.

Figuring out why I wasn't able to sleep ended up helping me tremendously. It took me a very long time—nearly thirty years, I believe, because my first baby was born a little over thirty years ago. When that happened, I should have been on top of the world. I enjoyed my position as a bassoonist in the Netherlands Philharmonic Orchestra. I was leading a successful life. I had a loving husband, a good income, and people who respected me for my skill and dedication. I adored my child and I was thrilled to be a mother. I should have been shouting my joy from the rooftops, but I didn't feel that way.

When I returned to work after my maternity leave was over, I wasn't able to sleep. From that day on, insomnia affected every aspect of my life. I became determined to solve this problem, not only for myself but for my family as well. Although, despite my best efforts, it would last well over twenty-five years.

With this book, my goal is to help you achieve your healing much faster than that. I went through this healing process all on my own. I had no mentor, no one who had already been through it to guide me. It is my hope that, with the help I'm offering here, you may be less resistant than I was to accepting some of the things your body is trying to tell you.

So, how is it for you? Do you ever feel lost? Like there's something wrong with you? I had those same feelings. I wanted to get rid of that negative view of myself with all my heart, and I tried to compensate for it by working very hard and doing things perfectly. I desperately wanted my parents to feel that big YES of acceptance for me in their hearts. Only then would I have felt that they were proud of me, and maybe even really loved me.

Maybe then, I thought, my parents would be able to put aside their own interests once in a while and participate in the world of their child, rather than attaching so much importance to whether they received their drinks on time or making sure they had time for their hobbies. But instead, everything had to be done exactly in accordance with the rules of the adults. That's how things were in those days.

I clearly remember that it felt like the house rules were much more important than I was. What did I know? I was like a blank slate, and having to obey their numerous rules restricted my development of a healthy feeling that I was okay as the person I was, that simply *being me* was enough. Feeling supported for who I was would have been much more effective than being continuously criticized.

I vividly remember how my father regularly said to my brother, "You are a nail in my coffin." To me, my parents often said, "Oh, Antoinetta, there's always something wrong with you. You always mess things up." Perhaps these are only words, but they aren't things that a parent should say to their children. For a child, everything is more intense, and they believe what they are told about themselves.

The messages I internalized about myself were: *You create too many problems. Everyone walks away from you. No one can stand to be around you.* And as the sweet little girl in need of parental acknowledgment that I was back then, how could I put those judgments about my character aside and lead my own happy life? Maybe there are children who can. I could not. I was adamant in my determination to refute all those criticisms and prove that I was better than what my parents thought of me. And that's exactly what I've been working toward my entire adult life as well.

If you are faced with a sleep disorder later in life, this often still has something to do with the messages you received about yourself during childhood. It's likely that there have been moments in your life that did not seem all that important at the time but that still form the foundation of how you feel about yourself now.

When I was in grade school, I always tried to come up with excuses for why I had to stop playing with my neighborhood friends in the late afternoons because I was expected to be home earlier than they were. I was never allowed to wear the "right" clothes, and I had an unfashionable hairstyle because my father preferred it that way, which only added to my sense that I didn't belong, a sense that has stayed with me for a long time.

Those feelings of self-doubt accompany you day in and day out when you interact with other children. They affect your ability to establish relationships and ultimately contaminate whatever sense you have of yourself. After all, if your parents hold such a mirror in front of you, then that is how you come to see yourself; you don't know any better. The mirror says, "I am not okay!" So, your sense of yourself is that you are not okay! When you are very young, your parents are like God to you. What they say is an absolute truth.

I felt insecure because of my parents' attitude toward me. I never developed a sense of being allowed to be myself, let alone of being proud of who I was. I thought that my "self" wasn't good enough and started compensating for that by trying to make self-improvements. I was constantly looking at others to see how they did things, how they behaved. I had no sense that it was okay for *me* to be *me* so I tried to change my behavior and live up to the conditions I thought would lead to approval.

This way of living doesn't enable you to develop a sense that *you* are *you* and that you have the right to be true to yourself. In other words, it prevents you from developing a *sense of self*. You are constantly working to ensure that you are included, that you count, because you're scared as hell of not being seen or heard.

You become preoccupied with doing things that make you feel a little bit better about yourself. You are constantly on the lookout for appreciation from your parents, peers, or authority figures. You want to see that smile of approval on their faces, because it makes you feel like you can escape their criticism, at least in this one instance.

In this way, without consciously realizing it, you're building the foundation for *a substitute sense of self*. Because the path to your natural self is blocked, this artificial way of sensing yourself through the approval of others gradually takes away the opportunity to develop a true sense of yourself.

One clearly recognizable symptom of a substitute sense of self is having a very strong urge to feel worthy at the end of the day. The urge is often so strong that you would do anything to get it.

Sleeping disorders can be the consequence of dependence on approval and needing to feel worthy.

Being able to attain your substitute sense of self depends on your ability to fulfill a number of conditions. This perceived necessity can make you very restless and nervous because you think you *have to* meet those conditions to get the approval you need. When you aren't in contact with your real self, you don't have an inner support system in place.

It becomes so important to meet those conditions because the feelings of worthiness you get creates a temporary psychological backbone that you cannot function without.

You may wonder where insomnia comes into play in this situation. Insomnia is something that demands your attention. It's a force of nature that's asking you to stop what you're doing and look at your life. Try to see insomnia as the knight who wants to save you from the clutches of this unhealthy way of living. This sleeping disorder is generated by your subconscious, and its task is to keep you from submitting to these self-destructive habits.

If your sole purpose is to meet conditions that you hope will lead to approval, you're not present in and to your own life. You're not aware of who you are, or even of your presence in your own body. You never learned to give yourself attention—except for harshly criticizing yourself for not being good enough in one way or another—because you are possessed by the need for outside approval and attention from others.

Sleeping issues can, therefore, be seen as a symptom of self-sabotage, or rather of *substitute sense of self sabotage*. You can look at self-sabotage as something you subconsciously yet purposely do (whether through action or inaction) that causes you to fail. At least, so it seems. Contrary to what you may think, this is, in essence, nature's way of trying to help you. Every being in existence needs to be itself. And when you're unable to sleep, nature is saying to you, *Pay attention! You are not yourself when you're chasing after approval.*

Insomnia prevents you from following the fictional script you're creating in your head when you imagine how things could (should!) work out differently for you if only you could manage to do this or that perfectly. It wants to show you that you are approaching things from an unhealthy motivation, that you are *not* doing things because you want to but because you depend on the approval you may get when you do them. You become so afraid that you'll fail to perform perfectly that your whole body reacts, even if you may not notice it. Except that you cannot sleep ...

You'd think that every time you did something right, you would sleep well, but the opposite is actually true. Inside you is a system that wants to help you become your true self. That system—I simply call it nature—wants you to understand that you're on the wrong track with the reasons for doing what you do.

Ultimately, every human being has the right to their own life, to develop their own personality and their own character. Every person has the right to enjoy their own talents and even their shortcomings. But parents who lack a sense of self often place a lot of importance on their children presenting themselves in certain ways. To generate a feeling of self-worth, these parents tend to either live vicariously through their children or use them as a means of gaining approval. At least that's how I explain what happened to me during my childhood.

Neither my father nor my mother had a healthy sense of self, and they did everything they could to achieve the social status they'd decided was necessary for them to feel worthy. They felt they were too good for the neighborhood we lived in, which meant that I wasn't allowed to play with the other children because "we are really much better than they are." This attitude, in hindsight, doesn't make sense at all, but in the 1950s and early 1960s, it was quite common to discriminate.

Being brought up this way left me with the feeling that I didn't belong. I remember that intense desire to belong to a group. As a child and young adult, I wished I was part of a working-class family because they seemed to be devoted to each other. I also imagined belonging to the Catholic Church, which I thought was very interesting: all these people coming together, connecting through rituals and shared belief. Our family didn't have close ties with anybody around us, which only served to feed my feelings of not belonging.

Childhood experiences and the conclusions you draw from them shape the way you see yourself and the world around you, which can have a dramatic impact on your ability to sleep.

You take it all with you when you go to bed at night.

What happens at night has everything to do with what you're chasing during the day and how dependent you are on the results you get. If you're satisfied with who and what you are, you're more likely to develop a natural sleeping pattern.

From this point of view, insomnia isn't the problem; it's a symptom of a deeper issue. Instead of trying to change how you sleep, you have to change how you feel about yourself. You have to dig into your past to be able to understand why you're suffering in the present: Were you able to develop a healthy sense of self early on in life, but some trauma or event interfered with that natural ability? Or were you like me and never developed a healthy sense of self in childhood?

Chapter 1

In the first case, you need to find your way back to sensing yourself as you did before. In the second case—whether it happened through neglect, being forced to live up to unrealistic expectations, or being used as a pawn so your parents/caregivers could live out their unfulfilled dreams through you—you need to learn how to get in touch with your real self. No matter how you came to this point in your life, the resulting need is the same, and learning (or relearning) to be your authentic self is the best medicine for helping you sleep.

Insomnia is nature's cue for you to find out what's going wrong in your life. It's an opportunity to correct the things that are working against your best interests and turn them around.

It would be better if nature were able to express its intention somewhat clearer, I agree. Being unable to sleep is upsetting, and it's not easy to understand why this is happening to you. But if you try to see things as I've described, it will help you look at your sleeping problems from a different angle.

If you can't sleep and you have no idea why, then you have to find the courage to look inside and ask yourself, *What's going wrong in my life? What am I doing wrong?* Here, your insomnia can be exactly the blessing you need to help you solve the underlying problems that are preventing you from living your life to the fullest. Eventually, you may even be grateful for your experience with insomnia because it ended up bringing you closer to yourself. Once you've gotten in touch with your real self, then you will sleep a lot better.

Tonight, before going to bed, stand in front of the mirror and look yourself in the eye. Ask yourself, *What am I actually doing? What do I hope to gain? Who am I really doing this for?* It's okay if you don't have the answers right away; it's okay if you're not even sure what part of your life these questions are aimed at. The point is to begin your inner quest for the truth behind your sleeplessness.

In the next chapter, we will look at what the root cause of your insomnia might be. We will also take the first step toward getting rid of it.

SUMMARY

1. Psycho-Emotional Stress Insomnia (PESI; see page 137) is nature's way of helping you get your life back on the right track. It's a type of self-sabotage that forces you to let go of the promise of a substitute sense of self so you can find your way back to your real self.

2. When you feel that you are not enough, that you have to pretend to be different because you're not allowed to express your authentic personality, then you don't feel acknowledged as your own person. This setup has an impact on the development of your sense of self during childhood, which has a long-lasting effect on your well-being throughout the rest of your life.

3. When you have a lack of sense of self, you think you have to work hard to get approval from others, which makes you feel worthy. It's a temporary state that functions as a substitute sense of self.

4. To earn approval and gain a substitute sense of self, you need to always do your best to accommodate the wishes of others and try to be how they want you

to be. Insomnia is born out of fear that you won't be able to do that.

5. Look into your past to find out what caused you to believe that you have to please others to feel worthy and what conditions you think you have to live up to.

6. To find out what's really motivating your actions, ask yourself, *Why do I do what I do?*

7. Once you've gotten in touch with your authentic self, you will sleep much better at night.

CHAPTER 2

What Your Self-Image Can Do to Your Sleep Cycle

*Consciously experience your body
to release your insomnia.*

Does chronic insomnia affect people who are comfortable in their own skin and secure in their sense of self? I don't think so! If you know who you are and what you want, this long-term sleep disorder won't haunt you unless something happens that throws you completely off balance: the death of a loved one, a gigantic setback in your career, a serious illness, or another such life-shattering event.

In this chapter, I will explain how the source of your sleeping problems may have taken root at a very early stage of your life. We are all formed by our environment and our upbringing. We live the way we were shaped during our formative years, and we sleep the way we live. This means that what happens in early childhood is indirectly responsible for the sleeping patterns we develop later in life.[1]

Children who grow up in a supportive environment have parents or other caregivers who give them the freedom to discover their true self and encourage them to feel good about who they are. Others of us who grow up with conditional regard are doomed to constantly earning approval over the course of our lives because we've never felt acknowledged and accepted as our own person.[2] How we deal with that situation will differ, depending on our individual temperament, character, and the way we learned to deal with our emotions.

Feeling like you don't belong creates a negative self-image because the message you receive is that you aren't good enough to be included. But feeling invisible can be a self-fulfilling prophecy—when you don't feel like you're being seen or heard or taken into consideration, it's a natural reaction to shrink in on yourself and not do anything to stand out. You may feel blocked from being able to express yourself, whether it's at home, at school, or at work. You may end up living on the sidelines, merely a spectator of the fun other people are having.

When I was young, I was haunted by that feeling of uneasiness with myself. I was eager to participate in activities with others, but I didn't feel up to it. One day, when I was about sixteen years old, I was standing on the beach looking out over the sea. I noticed a long pole rising up from the surface of the water. I imagined that the sea, instead of being full of water, was filled with people. I pictured myself sitting on that pole, removed from everyone around me and unable to reach any of them. The endlessness of this sea of people only increased my terrible sense of loneliness and isolation.

I desperately wanted to belong. To that end, I really wanted to wear trendy clothes and have a fashionable hairstyle. I thought that if I looked cool, it would help me be accepted by my peers. But my parents, particularly my father, thought the popular styles were all tacky and below our station.

In those days, girls preferred to wear their hair in ponytails with somewhat longer bangs. They also wore "rock 'n' roll stockings" (long red nylons), short skirts, and lots of makeup. Well, I certainly was not allowed any of that. After much begging and pleading, my father let me put my hair up in a ponytail, but he insisted on my bangs being very short. Way too short to be cool! I had to wear long skirts, and I got red socks instead of nylons, which I pulled up as high as possible the moment I was out of the door. Even though the length of my skirts helped to hide my socks, I still keenly felt the shortcomings in my appearance.

I hesitantly took to the streets each day, insecure with my fresh face, my short hair, and my too-long skirts. The negative judgment I passed on myself quickly preceded me. What do you think my schoolmates' reaction was? Would the other kids want to be my friends?

My parents deliberately did whatever they could to keep me from developing relationships with my peers, because they were all deemed to be not good enough. And sometimes they were even considered dangerous ...

My father did some volunteer work at a probation institution for young people who had been in prison. On occasion, boys from the institution would come to our home to see my father. Once, I made the mistake of going on a bicycle ride with one of them. The magnitude of that mistake was completely unclear to me until I came back. I don't recall whether my father physically hit me, but in my memory, he did. "The only thing those boys want from you is for you to lie on your back for them," he warned me in a threatening tone. That evening, after my parents left to visit the neighbors, I stood behind the front door for a couple hours with a hammer poised above my head, ready to attack. If that boy came back to rape me, I would smash his brains in. Eventually, I was too tired to stand there any longer, so I went to bed, but the fear was so real that I slept with the hammer under my pillow.

I spent my lonely childhood constantly wondering *why?* Why were other children allowed to play with each other? Why did I always have to come home so much sooner than they did? Why did I have to go to bed so early? Even my wish to play with the neighborhood children inconvenienced my parents. They wanted me to not make their lives more difficult than they already were.

My parents, like many parents, had their own agenda, and their substitute sense of self depended on the success of it. So yes, I was, in fact, more of a bother because I hindered their ability to succeed. It was impossible to get a sense from my mother that I meant something to her—that I was important to her, that she loved me, that she was proud of me.

Gradually, of course, I discovered what to do and how to behave to earn something that looked like love: approval—or at least the absence of disapproval. I did my best to improve on all those desired behaviors because their approval, especially my mother's, made me feel more valuable. There wasn't any room for me to be my own person.

Developing your sense of self should happen naturally when you're growing up. But instead, I learned to comply with my parents' wishes and perform in ways that pleased them.

Of course, like every child, there are times when you want to impress your parents: "Mum, Dad, look at me!" That's when you do your best to show them that you're good at something so they'll admire your skills. But if they're too busy with their own story, it becomes a hopeless task. They might even be jealous of your performance and resentful of your abilities. And if, for whatever reason, they're unable to give you that much-needed approval, their rejection pushes you to try even harder to win their appreciation. Eventually, the lack of acknowledgment and search for approval reaches the point where you identify with all the tasks you've set for yourself.

What's stressful about these tasks is that you become dependent on the results to feel worthy of other people's time and attention. Being unable to obtain that feeling of worthiness provokes anxiety, because it functions as an artificial substitute for your missing sense of self. On an intuitive level, without a healthy sense of self, you feel that you are not enough—that you aren't allowed to participate in life or contribute to the world around you. In other words, you feel like you don't matter.

This negative self-image makes you even more fanatical in your attempts to bring all these tasks to a good end. You're not living your own life because you've become a slave to fulfilling all these self-imposed conditions in the hope of being accepted and taken into account. The fear of failure is huge because it feels like your very existence is on the line, but beware: *this only takes place in your mind*. It is not a real threat; that fear you feel is based on conclusions you made as a child.

Now stop reading for a moment and take a few minutes to ask yourself whether you, too, are dependent on obtaining certain results from your actions. To detect this, there are many questions you can ask yourself: Do you always have to perform tasks to perfection? Do you find yourself overly upset when things don't go as planned? Do you always have to complete everything? Do you feel like criticism of your work is an attack on you as a person? Is your reaction to failure disproportionate to the actual effect it has on your life?

Perfectionism, workaholism, and the need for control are all symptoms of acting from the wrong type of motivation. Many people who put their work above their life don't do so from a sense of passion for what they're doing. Very often, they live that way to get a sense of self-worth. With that, they can then close each workday having gained the substitute sense of self that is essential for them to function.

Now you may think you would sleep like a log when you've done things to perfection, but that's not the reality. The strange thing is that this way of manufacturing feelings of worthiness doesn't even lead to being able to sleep well. Why? Because once you manage to reach that feeling, you (subconsciously) become afraid of losing it, along with the substitute sense of self it provides. You want to hold on to it at all cost. And that fear is what keeps you awake.

This whole pattern of living, though, is based on the fictitious belief that you need a substitute sense of self.

Instead of living your life on your own terms, all your energy is focused on meeting the conditions you think will make you feel worthy. What happens is that you're living on autopilot. You're following a program you learned when you were still a child. The fact that these choices were made unconsciously, and a very long time ago, makes it hard to find the thread that will guide you to the *why* of it all.

Yet, if you want a good night's sleep, it's essential for you to deepen your insight into your past, that you take a good look at what conclusions you came to about yourself earlier in life and what you felt you needed to do to survive. Perhaps fulfilling all those conditions worked in your favor when you were young, but they're no longer useful in your life *now*; in fact, they really may have become a burden.

Moreover, this autopilot that governs you keeps you away from real life—*your own* life. When you're so absorbed in the pursuit of all those conditions and performances, it's impossible not to become at least somewhat mentally and emotionally distorted. Spontaneous thoughts and feelings are snowed under because your heart and mind only have room for what will immediately contribute to your achieving success with these conditions.

The trick to beating insomnia is to find the way back to your real self before bedtime. But that's a lot easier said than done. You likely don't even know that you're not in touch with your self (anymore). To help you on your way, I've devised several steps to support this process of learning to sense your real self. The following exercises will get you started on that path and will continue to help you throughout the process.

First, you must learn to effectively become aware of your body as well as your existence in it. It encourages you to develop a direct relationship between your physical self and your mental self. This is the starting point of understanding and sensing that you don't need to achieve results or feel worthy to experience yourself. The objective of these mind/body awareness exercises is to get in tune with your physical presence and the ability it gives you to interact with your surroundings.[3]

Begin by simply noticing that you are present and in control of your body when you bend your knees. Observe how your muscles move when you put your foot down and shift your weight from side to side. Touch the wall and feel its texture against your fingertips. Stretch your hands out to either side and take note of all the sensations running through you as you spread your arms wide. It's important to start small and build from that foundation. Once you become comfortable with being present to the act of bending and moving your body, you can move on to the next exercises that incorporate your thoughts and your other senses.

Becoming aware of the fact that you can see, hear, smell, feel, and taste is another path to finding your way back to your real self before bedtime. When you really experience and use your senses consciously, you get physical confirmation that you are indeed experiencing the world through your body. You may have a negative self-image—thinking that something is wrong with you or feeling that you don't belong—but you do have a self, all the same. Even if you've never really noticed or focused on your real self, you can begin to do so through consciously experiencing your body. You have the same thing that every other person on earth has, but this body you inhabit is uniquely yours.

Your body allows you to interact with your environment and with the people around you. Having a body gives you the right to manifest yourself in this world. Your senses should be celebrated too. They help you navigate your world. They enable you to form your own tastes, preferences, and opinions. You can absolutely give yourself permission to express your own temperament, tendencies, and talents, regardless of how others might perceive you. Once that concept takes root, you will start to see the difference between earning a substitute sense of self through living up to the conditions you set for yourself and owning who and what you actually are *yourself*.

There are many ways you can become more aware of your body through your thoughts. For example, you can take a mental trip through your body, from your head to your toes, bringing your full awareness to each of your limbs. When you're in bed, it's common to not think about your body at all, unless you're uncomfortable or in pain. Take your legs for instance: even though they're such a large part of your body, you might completely forget about them once you're lying down. Now bring your thoughts into them—think about how they feel from the inside out. Think about all the things they allowed you to do throughout the course of the day. Bring your conscious mind into them and appreciate them fully. Know that they are both completely yours! Yours alone!

These mind/body awareness exercises may feel a bit awkward at first since it's something most people don't usually spend time on, but stick with them. Eventually they will feel natural to you as they unite your physical self with your psychological self. By bringing your thoughts and conscious awareness into all the parts of your physical form, you will learn to mindfully acknowledge that your body belongs to you, and to no one else. Then you will draw the conclusion that you have (and are) this body that is uniquely yours—that you live in it and through it. That fact alone means you have the right to exist as who you are. The fact that you exist gives you the right to live your own life and express your own heart and soul. Be done with performing tasks that only serve to please other people, because the feeling of worthiness you get from their approval is no longer a sufficient substitute for sensing your real self.

It's easy to take our bodies for granted, without giving thought or thanks to what they do for us every day. Experiencing your own body is a subtle matter. It's too easy for our bodies to remain outside our awareness because of all the loud stimuli we're constantly bombarded with in our modern culture. But even without the distractions of technology, news, and numerous sources of entertainment, you will notice that getting in touch with your body is still not that simple.

Yet it is an essential tool for helping you overcome your insomnia. It will lead you to the conscious realization that you do not have to be dependent on feelings of worthiness to function. You can stop worrying about meeting all the conditions that lead to outside approval, and you can finally let go of your negative self-image.

Try to sense your body now with conscious intent. Feel that you are your body and that your body is you. Know that you exist, that you already are. And know that no failure or critical judgment can ever take this away from you. Even during times when you feel bad about yourself, you still exist and you are enough just as you are. Acknowledging this and learning to truly believe it will allow you to put an end to being dependent on approval.

In Chapter 3, you will learn how to free yourself from negative self-judgments and what obstacles you might meet along the way. Even though this may not seem like it's directly related to your insomnia, trust that it is the *right* path to getting a good night's sleep.

SUMMARY

1. Sleep is affected by the healthiness of your sense of self.
2. Your sense of self is shaped by the environment you grew up in.
3. You may have grown up learning to seek approval to gain validation.
4. The fear of failing to meet expectations causes severe stress and insomnia when you lack a sense of self.
5. When you lack a sense of self, you may feel that you're not enough—that you're not allowed to participate in life or contribute to the world around you.
6. To beat insomnia, take the time to center yourself before bedtime. Bring awareness to your body and your senses.
7. Having (and being) a body gives you the right to manifest yourself in this world.
8. Practice the mind/body awareness exercises at the end of this chapter regularly.

CHAPTER 3

Changing Your Behavior

Stop overcompensating for your feelings of inadequacy.

If you want natural, healthy sleep, it's important to change your negative self-image. This includes putting a stop to all reactions you have toward yourself, which can sometimes be extreme. These behaviors and inner thoughts may be intended to help refute that negative view of yourself, but by taking this negative self-image seriously, this reactivity is actually reinforcing it.

Getting a good night's sleep calls for a change in your behavior and your attitude. Sleeping is like breathing; if it doesn't come naturally, something is preventing it from happening. If your ability to sleep isn't caused by outside factors, it's coming from within you, and only you can change it.

In this chapter, we'll talk about reconditioning yourself. But before starting this process, you should first thoroughly examine your motivation for wanting better sleep, beyond the obvious physical need for rest. Ask yourself, *Am I absolutely sure my reason for wanting to be well rested isn't based on the unhealthy motivation of being in better shape for seeking approval?* What you discover may surprise you.

If you want to make a big leap in improving your sleep, you need to make adjustments not only to your outward behavior but also to your behavior toward yourself. You have to change your whole way of thinking about yourself because this change in attitude eventually leads to feeling differently about yourself, your life, and your place in the world. In other words, you have to recondition yourself. Keep in mind that this is a life-changing journey and you shouldn't expect perfection; relapse is inevitable when changing your behavior. Be gentle with yourself when it happens and know that it's a normal part of the process.

My process started years ago, with a dream. I was going through many different therapies, eager to find one that would work. I tried every possible method I came across that might get rid of my insomnia: talk therapy with a psychologist, neuro-linguistic programming (NLP),[1] eye movement desensitization and reprocessing treatment (EMDR),[2] meditation, yoga, hypnotherapy, and more. I'd hoped to find one that would fix whatever it was that kept me from sleeping every night. But none of them did. At least, not at that time.[*]

---

[*] In hindsight, I realize that some of these therapies are great tools, but I wasn't ready for them at that time. I hadn't laid the necessary groundwork for them to help me. Years later, in the advanced stages of my healing process, using EMDR[3] in conjunction with Neurological Integration System (NIS)[4] proved to be extremely effective.

Chapter 3

Luckily, I had a revelation in the form of the following dream:

> *A gigantic featherless bird soared high above me. It looked like an elongated plucked chicken. I was able to spot all the bumps on its skin, with little hairs sticking out where its feathers should be. I was standing in a forest, and the bird cast a huge shadow over the beautiful flowers and plants surrounding me. I called it the ugly bird—it was far from pleasant to look at—but, for some reason, I identified with that big unsightly beast.*

A sunbeam fell like a spotlight on a beautiful little bird, pulling my attention away from the monster above. The little bird sat peacefully on an inviting mossy stone at the edge of a shiny pond. The weather was fantastic, and the bees were happily buzzing about the flowers at the water's edge. The little bird had the most beautiful colors: a deep blue body with shiny golden wings and an ample orange tail. It looked like a brightly colored nightingale.

That dream and the meaning it held has stayed with me ever since. Because of this dream, I started to wonder what my life was all about. Why did I identify with that great ugly creature? Why did I want nothing to do with that pretty little bird?

I began to realize that, in my mind, I was living way beyond my natural human proportions. I wanted *too much*; my aspirations were far too big. Why was that? Because I assumed that this was necessary for me to be seen and heard. Through working very hard, I wanted to prove that I

How to Overcome Insomnia All by Yourself

had value, that I was allowed to exist and that I was not the pitiful little girl I felt I was in the eyes of my parents.

The ugly bird was the symbol for all the tasks that I had (unconsciously) set for myself so that I could prove my parents wrong and earn my substitute sense of self. The beautiful little bird was me in real size. The message this dream left me with was that I needed to turn that ugly bird into the little nightingale. At the same time, the nightingale seemed so small and insignificant that I didn't want to go through that transformation at all. For a long time to come, I preferred to stay the big ugly bird that cast a dark shadow over everything.

Letting go of the artificial self that I'd spent my life cultivating and maintaining was scary. But if I didn't want the beauty of the world to pass me by unnoticed, if I wanted any chance to enjoy life, I would have to turn my *will* and my *heart* around. I would have to *truly want* to make that my reality. I would have to abandon those demanding and fictitious conditions I struggled to meet every day. I would have to recondition myself.

Now please ask yourself how this resonates with you. What is the blueprint of your existence? What does the bigger picture of your life look like in your mind? What makes you get out of bed in the morning? Why do you do the things you do?

If the answers to these questions show that you have set yourself the impossible task of proving to your loved ones that you are worthy of their love and attention, then you need to realize that you already *are* and that you shouldn't have to prove your value to them. To be able to make that giant leap in self-perception, you must first decide to recondition yourself. By doing so, you will change your

32   C   Antoinetta Vogels

motivation for doing things, which will ultimately lead to a healthier sleeping pattern.

Reconditioning, what is that exactly? It sounds like a formidable word, but you can do it on your own. It means that you have to teach yourself to think differently. You've built up a lot of habits since childhood that live deep under the surface of your awareness. And it is precisely those habits that you need to review and, if necessary, change.

People are creatures of habit. And as I'm sure you've discovered when trying to break habits in the past, some are very entrenched and quite difficult to change. To visualize this, I tend to compare the human brain to a tree without leaves. Imagine a fruit tree in winter: the branches are bare, and you can clearly see its shape. If one branch is in the way of another, you can grab a saw and cut it off. That way, you give the tree more space for balanced growth so that it can produce more fruit in the spring.

Unfortunately, it's not possible to perform this pruning process with our brains. We can't see the map of our intertwining neurological pathways or trim and shape them as we'd like to. But what you can do is imagine your mind as a landscape: think of what the specific areas look like, and make a drawing of them. Then you can come up with certain conclusions, such as *I think the vegetation may be a little too dense in this area.* Or: *This field is probably too empty; maybe I should try to grow some bushes there.* In this way, you can form a visual map of how you are made.

Changing your own behavior is a process that takes time. After all, it has also taken a long time to develop your habits and automatic reactions/behaviors. You can't change them from one day to the next. You can compare this process to cleaning up a garden that has grown wild, and this is where the mind map you drew comes in handy. Pinpoint the areas that need sprucing up. You may want to start by pulling the weeds. Next, give it some shape by carving a path and determining the places you want to plant seeds and flowers.

Just like in a real garden, when you recondition yourself, you have to perform continuous maintenance on the work that's already been done. We all know how stubborn weeds are, and bad habits tend to grow back just as tenaciously. To some extent, this is bound to happen. The changes you're making are so big that you can't avoid falling back into old habits. But relapse can be minimized by not making this reconditioning process an isolated activity. Try to see this as a lifestyle change. You will benefit greatly from continuously going back to what you've already done. You can work on yourself little by little every day, for a few minutes or half an hour or even two hours. Of course, we all have different demands on our time, but it's important to set some aside for yourself every day. The more time you're able to dedicate to this process, the faster you'll solve your sleeping problems.

So, how do you proceed to recondition yourself and change your behavior? You begin by looking at who you are right now. Be utterly honest with yourself. Don't try to sugarcoat it or present yourself as more agreeable than you are. Don't justify your behavior with obvious or plausible excuses that, on an honest level, have nothing to do with it. Being honest with yourself is essential for this process to succeed.

Remember the exercise from Chapter 2, geared toward learning to experience your own body, become aware of your senses, and strengthen the connection between your mind and your body. You want to continue using those exercises to learn to experience yourself from the inside out. The feeling that you "are" already, without having to achieve results or gain the appreciation of others, is called being grounded in yourself. *You already are.* You have the right to be just as you are, purely because you exist. This is the sensation you need to nurture and return to over and over.

But keep in mind that this may be new for you, so it's important to repeat this exercise regularly: just find an easily accessible touchstone (the wall, your desk, the arm of your chair) and reach for it again and again to create that awareness: *I feel, so I am.*

Here's another exercise to add to your daily practice: being in the Here and Now. Take a good look around. Pay attention to your immediate surroundings and try to remind yourself, *I'm not in the past. I am in the Here and Now.* Try to understand that all those conditions you think you have to live up to are rooted in problems from the past. Living up to these conditions is your subconscious mind's way of trying to solve these problems in the present. The discrepancy in time alone dooms these attempts to failure. When you can see that what you're doing is motivated by issues from your past, you have to seize that moment to experience your true present-day reality: *I am in the Here and Now.*

Ask yourself what this reality looks like and describe it out loud to yourself. For example, is there a clear danger causing your insomnia? Is there a lion next to your bed? Does it want to eat you? Or is there an elephant on the porch trying to squeeze its way into your house? Probably not! The threat isn't real; it's caused by your perception of having to live up to conditions that exist only in your mind.

Now that you know this, you can form your own independent opinion about these conditions. Quiet any inner voices that don't belong to your true self and ask, *What should I do now that I know I don't need to fulfill these conditions? Who am I, based on my real reality and not in relation to anyone else? What kind of person am I?* And once you have taken these steps toward truly seeing yourself, then you'll be able to look around and see other people as they truly are.

For me, becoming truly aware that other people were actually other people took place in a specific setting. It struck me for the first time when I was driving. I used to be quite afraid of causing an accident. But one day, I suddenly realized that it wasn't just up to me—all the other drivers also had eyes in their heads and the ability to react to situations. It was just as much their responsibility to be alert to their surroundings as it was mine. Those other drivers most likely felt the need to do whatever they could to prevent a collision too. In other words, *these other people were able to see me.* So, it was not up to me alone to keep an eye on all the other cars around me and prevent an accident from happening.

That insight into reality ties back to my childhood. I had always felt that it was my fault if something went wrong. If there was a fight, if happy hour was disturbed, if anything didn't go the way it was supposed to go, I was always the one to blame. I held on to that idea throughout most of my life. But as soon as I began to realize I wasn't always the one at fault, I started to see others for who they are, as their own unique person.

Everyone has their own goals, and the motivation behind those goals can be either healthy or unhealthy.

We all have our own hopes and dreams, and others pursue things you don't know anything about. Every person has the right to go through their own developmental phases, at their own pace. And each one of us has to solve our lack of insight and maturation for ourselves. We all live in individual bubbles and see the world through a unique lens of perception. Nobody has the power to pull you out of your own mindset and say, "You have to live exactly as *I* live in *my* bubble." Your life belongs to you, and you can walk your own path.

Now here is that crucial question: Why are you so desperate to sleep? Not wanting to be so tired all the time is a first and obvious reason, of course. But ask yourself *why* you want to sleep well. What was it that made you get out of bed this morning? What was the underlying purpose of what you did today? It could be that you're trying to solve your sleeping issues precisely to be better able to realize your hidden goal, the real reason preventing you from sleeping in the first place. This motivation is one that needs to be understood and intercepted. Only then can your hidden goal be eliminated and turned into a healthy objective.

It's important to understand that your hidden goal is stopping you from living your life for yourself because you're so focused on proving that you have value. Take a good look at how you truly see others: Are they nothing more to you than a means to an end or obstacles to overcome on the way to your sacred goal? Don't feel bad if this resonates with you; it's not because you're a bad person.

If you can truly see others and yourself as individual beings who exist unconditionally, you can let go of the need for a substitute sense of self. Then, everything you do will really be about what you're doing, without any hidden agenda or drive to feel worthy.

Free yourself from being dependent on results. Get to the point where you clean your kitchen because you want a nice place to cook, rather than wanting to get approval and feel good about your clean kitchen. And if you're pursuing your chosen career because your heart is fully in it—not because you want to make your father proud—you will be able to sleep better at night.

Make your way through the jungle of change, and by the time you arrive at the other side of the forest, you'll know that it was well worth the effort. You'll be able to fully participate in life and do things because it's what you want or because it needs to be done. You will use your talents and energy to make a better life and a better world. And when you become your authentic self, healthy sleep becomes natural too. All that is possible when you become emotionally independent.

Now that you've reached the end of this chapter, please take some time to consider what you can do to become your real self. How can you step out of the delusion of the ugly bird and accept the tiny nightingale that embodies the beauty that lives inside you? Change the image of the birds to anything that suits you better—maybe it's fish, bears, or dogs. Think of any images that feel right for you and play that scenario out in your mind.

To sleep better, you must check to see if you're perhaps demanding too much from yourself and ask why that would be. By becoming aware of your previously subconscious motives, you open up the opportunity to do things differently. Everything comes down to the question of why you do what you do.

In the next chapter, we will look at how you can adjust your motivation to stay true to yourself and sleep better.

SUMMARY

1. To sleep better, you need to change your motivation and your perception of yourself. Making those changes involves reconditioning your mind.
2. Assess how real you feel right now. Be honest with yourself about your behavior and motives.
3. Relapse is bound to happen. Just keep bringing awareness to your true self and continue with the reconditioning process.
4. When you let go of your need for a substitute sense of self, you will see others and yourself as individual beings who have the right to exist unconditionally.
5. When you use your life to gain other people's approval, you give them power over you, and you miss out on living your own life.
6. Accepting your limitations will help you sleep better.
7. Think of an image you resonate with to describe yourself when you're chasing your substitute sense of self. Create a counterbalance to this image to represent your true self. Compare these two images and use them to investigate your motivations when you're making decisions.

Sonnet 27

Weary with toil, I haste me to my bed,
The dear repose for limbs with travel tired;
But then begins a journey in my head,
To work my mind, when body's work's expired:
For then my thoughts (from far where I abide)
Intend a zealous pilgrimage to thee,
And keep my drooping eyelids open wide,
Looking on darkness which the blind do see:
Save that my soul's imaginary sight
Presents thy shadow to my sightless view,
Which, like a jewel hung in ghastly night,
Makes black night beauteous and her old face new.
Lo, thus, by day my limbs, by night my mind,
For thee, and for myself, no quiet find.

–William Shakespeare

CHAPTER 4

Sleepless Nights and Your Daily Motivation

The choices you make during the day
determine how you sleep at night.

Perhaps you're like I was, and you've become so accustomed to not sleeping well that you tend to forget it's a serious problem. You may not even consider that there's a clear explanation for why you can't sleep.

Sleeping problems occur mostly at night. Therefore, it's smart to first investigate your sleep environment.[1] Examine whether anything in your surroundings or circumstances is potentially supporting your sleep or what might be playing a role in your insomnia.[2] Maybe your pillow is too high or too dense? Perhaps it causes neck pain that keeps you up all night as you try to find a better sleeping position. It could be that your mattress is uncomfortable. Or maybe your partner snores or talks in their sleep.

There's plenty of literature about what factors can disturb your sleep and what practical adjustments you can make to alleviate them. Here are a few common suggestions: Take time to relax before going to bed. Turn off or put away all electronic devices, such as your TV and smartphone, at least thirty minutes before you climb into bed. Try to wake up and go to bed at the same time every day.[3]

But what if the main cause of your insomnia can't be solved with a new bed or a white noise machine? What if you need to change your lifestyle? Hidden in the subconscious territory of your psyche, there may be a process going on that determines whether or not you'll get a good night's sleep. A process that aims at the realization of a strategy you developed early in life but that still *motivates* your daily doing and thinking.

Some cause-and-effect situations are easy to recognize because they play out in the open. After strenuous physical exercise, whether it's weight training, dance class, a long walk along the beach, or an exhausting bicycle ride, your body is tired and you're more likely to sleep well.

Mental work creates a different kind of fatigue. Now it's your brain, eyes, ears, and maybe even your voice that have been exerted. Your mind is stimulated after this kind of workout, and it needs some time to return to its natural, relaxed state. For most people, it's difficult to fall asleep when the mind has been active but the body has not, especially if your muscles are stiff from hours of sitting in the same position. After a long day of mental work, it's best to plan downtime that includes light stretching before going to bed.

Fatigue also occurs as a result of emotions. Intense emotional experiences may leave you feeling depleted. Sometimes emotional fatigue can lead to a night of deep, refreshing sleep, sometimes not—much depends on the nature of these emotions and how well you've processed them.

Psychological stress can have a negative impact on your sleeping pattern as well, causing what I call *psycho-emotional stress insomnia* (PESI).*

Experiencing psychological stress is quite disconcerting, especially because you're not always aware of it. You may feel tension but can't figure out where it's coming from. Sometimes this tension manifests in your neck or your back, sometimes it's in your legs, or you feel it in your stomach. In my case, I felt it in the back of my skull. To recognize the sensation, I described it as feeling as if my sleeping scales were upended.

At times my insomnia would take me by complete surprise, but there were some nights I'd anticipate that I wouldn't be able to fall asleep. On those nights, something inside me felt activated. I was totally alert and ready to jump out of bed at any moment. Maybe it was adrenaline, or maybe something else. Human bodies are complex, and, unfortunately, I don't have insight into the potential physical, chemical, or electrical imbalances that may have contributed to my insomnia. I can only say how I experienced it.

Psychological stress was chronically present in my life; I was scared to death of being unable to gain that substitute sense of self I thought I needed. This is how I came to explain

---

* See Appendix B for more information on Psycho-Emotional Stress Insomnia (PESI).

my condition to myself to get a grip on it. There weren't any signs indicating where I could go to find out what was really going on. But by taking a good look inside, I concluded that I was terrified of not living up to the specific conditions that would lead to approval and allow me to feel worthy. My perception that living up to those conditions was an absolute must turned out to be my major source of stress and anxiety.

Being under chronic psychological stress means that you are under perpetual mental and emotional pressure, often without knowing why. If your goal is to prove to others (and to yourself) that their negative image of you is wrong, it causes tremendous stress. Living under the burden of such an unattainable (hidden) goal colors your motivation and seriously impacts your sleep.

> Motivation is the engine that drives behavior.
> Healthy motivation doesn't obstruct a good
> night's sleep; unhealthy motivation does!
> It's up to you to find out whether your motivation
> to do or avoid something is healthy or not.

Healthy motivation means that you do what you do because it benefits you, because it has to be done, or because you like to do it. Healthy motivation goes hand in hand with a healthy sense of self. When you know you're enough as who you are, you don't need to prove yourself to anyone, so your motivation stays on point.

Unhealthy motivation indicates that you have a hidden agenda, which is rooted in the need to compensate for a lack of sense of self. Although you may partly do what you do because it needs to be done, you also still do things to feel good about yourself.

Taking all this into consideration, we can say that insomnia is essentially caused by unhealthy motivation, which implies a lack of sense of self. Restoring your sense of self is the remedy. If you want to sleep better, it's a matter of identifying the nature of your motivation. One way to do that is by measuring the degree of intensity of your emotions.

The process of chasing a goal that's perceived to provide a feeling of having permission to exist is loaded with great fear and psychological stress. Emotions are typically more intense than they would be under normal circumstances. If you can take a step back and examine the way you react to situations, you'll be in the position to identify which emotions are out of balance. The next step is to find out which situations are likely to trigger these acute flare-ups of intense emotions so you know what adjustments you need to make.

When reconditioning yourself, it's necessary to address the subconscious part of your behavior. The reactions you tend to produce when living on autopilot need to be questioned and then altered based on your *own* opinion. Once you're able to recognize your ulterior motive, you've opened the door to a paradigm shift toward healthy motivation.

With a healthy sense of self, you sleep better
because you do things for the direct, obvious reason.
You don't depend on approval or the outcome
of your actions for your sense of self-worth.

Even though I loved music, I chose to be a professional musician for the wrong reason. My decision was primarily based on my hope of earning my mother's acknowledgment, appreciation, and admiration. Above all, I saw my mother's deep regard for people who were skilled at playing music. So I thought, *If I become an accomplished musician like those people she admires, I'll finally be worthy of her appreciation and true love.*

I chose to learn to play the bassoon—the bass of the woodwinds. It's known as quite a stubborn instrument that comes with an added difficulty of having to build your own reeds by hand—an art in and of itself. And after only three weeks, it became clear to me that it was going to be a struggle. I should have said then and there, "No way! That's not for me!" But instead, I went with my mother to her amateur orchestra in the hopes of making her proud. A few years later, I enrolled in the Royal Conservatory of Music—digging myself even deeper into it.

After regularly assisting in various orchestras, I landed a permanent position in The Netherlands Philharmonic Orchestra. For the onlooker, I seemed successful, but I knew what price I was paying: anxiety, fear, and working relentlessly. I practiced and practiced like crazy, but it didn't bring the desired praise, and my mother's attitude toward me didn't change. So, I started learning other instruments, looking to achieve more glory by trying to be a musical octopus. I was secretly in awe of people who were well versed in so many instruments, and I wanted to be like them. I tried singing, the saxophone, the piano, and then added the violin and the flute to my growing repertoire. I tried everything. But it wasn't so much about *what* I did but *why* I did it—what I truly wanted to achieve. I'd internalized the self-image that I wasn't enough, and I wanted to prove that I was worth the attention and admiration of others.

In the process, I completely fragmented my musical energy and felt as if I hadn't accomplished anything. In the orchestra, I functioned reasonably well, but at the expense of myself and my own life. There were many ways my body tried to tell me something was wrong. For example, after studying hard to become a successful singer, I got a very bad cold the day before my first concert. My voice was unusable and so the event could not go on. While I now know that this is a typical case of self-sabotage* subconsciously undermining my unhealthy motivation, I had no idea about that in those days. In fact, I didn't consider these truths until I hit my mid-thirties, when I became ill with hepatitis, probably due to chronic exhaustion.

Having an illness taught me that I had been hugely overextending myself. Not so much because of my multiple endeavors or the long days of hard work, but because of the psycho-emotional burden of desperately needing to be successful that undermined me.

Before the birth of my daughter, I was able to get away with functioning under unhealthy motivation, but once I was a mom, it kept me from getting a restful night's sleep for years. Any insight that the seemingly simple desire to feel worthy was part of a complex psycho-emotional constellation was still missing and, therefore, kept me hostage for far too long.

So, how do you find out what the nature of your motivation and the status of your sense of self is?

A reliable benchmark to find out whether or not your motivation is healthy is to monitor the intensity of your emotions. When something goes wrong, do your emotions

---

* See Appendix C for more information about self-sabotage as it relates to the sabotage of the substitute sense of self.

run haywire? Are you angry a lot? Does your level of frustration regularly reach the point that you want to break something or beat up everybody around you? Do you continuously yell at your siblings, pets, kids, or spouse? Do you think about harming yourself or others? If you answered yes to any of these questions, chances are your default emotional patterns are programmed to make you feel worthy so you can negate your negative self-image.

Here are a few examples to illustrate this. If you find any of these scenarios difficult to relate to, try to focus on the emotional aspects. We all come from different backgrounds and react differently to things, so just do your best to picture yourself in each situation.

1. Imagine that you made an extravagant salad using the finest toppings, hoping to impress your dinner guests. When the moment comes to sit down together, you catch your spouse picking all the tasty ingredients out of the serving dish with his fingers. Instead of being mildly annoyed and quietly scolding him, you completely lose it: you grab the plate of croquettes and throw them one by one into the salad, yelling at him that he's ruined everything. The intensity of this reaction shows that your emotion is not in accordance with the actual event. Your spouse may have bad manners, but his behavior didn't cause a catastrophe.

What could be the real reason for your fury?

You didn't organize this lunch to have a good time with your guests; rather, you were subconsciously angling for their approval to give you a feeling of worthiness. Your spouse's embarrassing behavior thwarted that goal, and that's what caused your furious response.

2. Suppose you just finished mopping the floor and your roommate comes in wearing muddy boots. Of course, having your hard work negated is irritating, but if you go nuts and sling insults at him like he's the worst person on earth, the intensity of your emotion may reveal that there's something else going on. It's more than just the fact that your time and effort were wasted because your roommate was inconsiderate and didn't take his shoes off before coming inside.

What could be really at play?

"If I don't have this floor clean by the time my father comes to visit, he'll be annoyed and blame me for it. I need to do my best to keep him in a good mood so I can feel good about myself."

3. Picture your child coming home with a bad report card, and you take it as a personal insult. You go to great lengths to tell her how stupid she is, and that she'll never amount to anything. And how can it be possible that she's not able to get good grades when you put in so much effort to ensure she does her homework on time? Yes, good grades are better than bad ones, but can you see how this reaction is about something else and not really about what's important for your child?

What could be the underlying cause for your rage?

Maybe you're afraid that your own parents or your child's teacher will criticize the way you're raising your kid. Or you hate seeing a bad report card because it means you'll have to spend more time tutoring your child instead of focusing on things that will lead to approval at work.

4. Imagine you just baked a beautiful cake. As you admire it from across the room, your dog jumps on the table and gobbles up your masterpiece. This may seem like a legitimate reason to be upset and punish your dog. Of course it's an irritating situation, but the intensity of your emotions and the way you react to your dog are indicative of the nature of your motivation.

What could be behind your reaction?

If your motivation for making the cake was healthy, your annoyance is directly related to the bad behavior of your dog and the loss of your time, effort, and ingredients. However, if you made the cake with the intention of using it to earn approval, your motivation is unhealthy. You perceive the loss as something much greater, which could cause you to fly into a rage or sink into despair.

A certain degree of frustration is appropriate in each of these examples, but none of them are exactly the end of the world. Can you think of some situations in your own life where your reaction was disproportionate to the event that caused it? If you find that the intensity of your emotions can sometimes be a bit too high, it may be time to start looking within. Introspection is the only way to find out why you react the way you do.

Chapter 4

Being extremely attached to the results of your actions or behavior can disrupt your ability to sleep. Ask yourself, *What do I really dread if I fail to do this or that in a specific way or within a specific time frame?* If the consequence is relatively minor, there could be something else behind the importance you're attaching to the situation. Anger is used to mask fear, so if you often find yourself feeling angry, ask yourself, *What exactly am I so afraid of that can make me so angry?*

Keep an eye on how you react to things. Of course, that's easier said than done. It's easy to forget to prioritize the care of your emotions in the course of daily life. But with practice and determination, you can get it done. And if you forget to evaluate yourself in the moment or in the immediate aftermath of an event, you can always look at your behavior or reaction in retrospect: "Even though my reaction was quite fierce, it was justified in light of the event that triggered it." Or maybe just the opposite: "Well, the emotions that bubbled up when my friend told me we might have to cancel our plans for the weekend were greatly exaggerated. What could be behind that?"

This way, you can map your own emotions and determine if your reactions stem from healthy or unhealthy motivation. This exercise will provide you with a lot of information about the quality of your sense of self.

In the previous chapters, we addressed how a negative self-image is formed early in life due to a child's dysfunctional relationship with their parents or other caregivers. The result is a lack of sense of self, which causes unhealthy motivation. With this in mind, ask yourself, *Was I truly seen and allowed to be myself when I was growing up? Did I get the attention that I needed? Did I have to work hard to be noticed? Did I feel unsafe at home or at school? Was I ever neglected or mistreated? Did I feel unconditionally loved?* Your answers to these questions will shed light on why you might have developed a hidden agenda for your actions or behaviors.

In the next chapter we'll take a closer look at why some people have a healthy motivation and others do not. We'll also find out what you can do to correct unhealthy motivation.

SUMMARY

1. Address all the physical elements in your sleep environment. Make sure it's dark, cool, quiet, and comfortable enough to fall asleep.

2. Plan downtime that includes light stretching before going to bed. Turn off all electronic devices, such as your TV and smartphone, at least thirty minutes before your climb into bed.

3. The quality of your sense of self determines the nature of your motivation, which influences how you sleep.

4. Motivation is the engine that drives behavior. Healthy motivation doesn't obstruct a good night's sleep; unhealthy motivation does! It's up to you to find out whether your motivation to do or avoid something is healthy or not.

5. Study your behavior and discover what could be the psycho-emotional stressors that are leading to your sleeping problems.

6. A reliable benchmark for finding out whether or not your motivation is healthy is to monitor the intensity of your emotions.
7. When it comes from a place of unhealthy motivation, extreme anger is caused by the fear and frustration of not being able to achieve a feeling of worthiness. Anger, fear, and sleep don't go together well.

CHAPTER 5

How Parental Mirroring Affects Your Sense of Self

Being yourself leads to getting a good night's sleep!

Our quality of life is for a large part determined by how well we sleep. Generally speaking, some days may be better than others, but one thing is certain: if you feel well rested, you're more likely to start the day with a positive attitude. Things are different when you have insomnia. Not only do you suffer at night but you're painfully reminded of your problem during the day as well.

You're lying there, staring at the ceiling night after night. Your eyes are unbearably tired from being kept open. Sometimes you squeeze them shut, pretending you're sleeping to ease the dread of facing yet another sleepless night. You toss and turn, trying to find the most comfortable position, throwing off the blankets, then pulling them back on. You're shivering some moments only to be covered with sweat the next. As the alarm clock counts down the hours that are left until you have to get up, you're haunted by the question: "Will I be able to sleep at all tonight?"

Filled with thoughts of what tomorrow holds, your anxiety grows: maybe there's an important meeting at work or you have to drive your carpool. Whatever responsibility is waiting the next morning is going to be that much more difficult if you can't get to sleep now.

Only those of us who have personally gone through the disheartening sensation of starting another day with hardly any sleep can truly resonate with this scenario. Even your loved ones have no idea how much you struggle with the resulting lack of energy and how much of yourself you're forced to put on the backburner because of it. The true toll of insomnia is that you're not allowed to participate fully in life!

When you don't have the vitality to do more than the bare minimum for yourself, making plans is no longer within your reach. Facing the responsibility of committing to anything feels daunting because you can't count on having enough energy to follow through. Sleeping problems dampen your desire to join in activities, even in those you normally enjoy most. Your lack of interest can eventually affect your relationships and lead to loneliness.

So how do you unravel the enigma of your sleeping problem?

The point of view I approach this topic from alternates between that of a parent and that of a child. Every parent has been a child and still carries that child within. And every child has the potential to become a parent or an educator and pass along what they learned when they were growing up. If you don't have children or don't plan on becoming a parent, it's still helpful to consider both viewpoints to get insight into your own childhood conclusions and the potential reasons behind them.

The development of healthy motivation depends on the way parents* relate to their child. Do they really see the child as being their own unique individual instead of as an extension of themselves? During childhood, a constellation of elements is put in place that determines susceptibility to insomnia later in life.

Why do some children automatically end up with a healthy sense of self while others don't? Unless they make a conscious decision to do things differently, parents/ caregivers tend to mirror children the way their parents/ caregivers mirrored them. The way an adult mirrors a child is influenced by their own childhood experiences, and unfinished business can be passed down from generation to generation. On your quest to solve your sleeping problem, gaining insight into the messages you received about yourself at an early age, regardless of where they came from, can be quite revealing.

Parental mirroring begins immediately after birth. Without being aware of it, a caregiver emits verbal and nonverbal messages about their child, which are picked up and internalized by this child. These messages reveal the parents' state of mind, their emotional involvement, and what their child means to them.

---

* Parents obviously have a major effect on their children, but caregivers, teachers, authority figures, and other influential adults can impact a child's development as well. When I talk about parents, I'm also generally referring to these other important adults.

Parents are often still very focused on whatever is playing out in their own lives. They may have personal problems or a demanding job. Their dependency on living up to conditions and getting approval could result in a situation where they never have the time or the peace of mind to focus on their child. But it's necessary for parents to pay sincere attention to their child during this time and cultivate a wholesome mutual understanding and appreciation. This lack of true involvement falls under the category of emotional neglect, which is a serious shortcoming in child-rearing. The consequences of that neglect can be drastic, and the child may end up with a negative self-image that can lead to insomnia.[1]

In addition, when parents lack a sense of themselves, they tend to force their child to behave and develop in ways that meet their own needs, insisting on the least amount of disruption within the family. They may try to minimize the impact their child has on their lives to better cope with their own problems.

But children want to feel loved and need to know that they matter to the important adults in their lives. They need to *be seen and heard* and have their existence confirmed.[2] Most parents have good intentions, but the complexity of life tends to blur the lines between what's best for the child and what's best for the parent. In the course of daily life, parents can unintentionally overlook their child's need for validation. But if the parents routinely fail to provide acknowledgment, an unhealthy idea will form in the child's heart and mind: "I'm not good enough as myself. I have to be different to win my parents' approval." The child will continuously try to find ways to please the parents. "What can I do to get that smile from my mother or father that makes me feel accepted?" becomes their main quest in life.

This strategy to get their parents' approval leads to behavioral changes that can go against their own nature. Parents don't usually change, and therefore, the need for approval doesn't change either, which only makes the child more determined to perfect the behavior *they know their parents want from them*.

Ultimately, this strategy is at the core of unhealthy motivation. When you aren't encouraged to be yourself, and your parents/caregivers don't facilitate your process of manifesting your own nature, you don't develop a sense of self. The void where your sense of self ought to be is instead filled by the need for approval.

Unhealthy motivation aims at scoring approval, and its only purpose is to make you feel worthy.

What does life look like when we act from unhealthy motivation? Chances are we become control freaks. Otherwise, our chance for gaining approval is at risk.

When sleeping well is something that gets you approval, as it was for me, the need for control can be apparent when it comes to your sleeping circumstances. Maybe you construct a ritual around your bedtime and have become dependent on meeting all those requirements. This dependency limits the freedom of your sleeping partner, if you have one.

Just as with a healthy relationship, when the period of infatuation is over, conflicts and annoyances are hiding around every corner as you try to adjust to each other's differences. You want the window open; your partner wants it closed. You just landed a great job, but your partner wants to move to another city to pursue their dreams. Considerations about who gets their way (or how much either of you is willing to sacrifice) becomes part of your daily routine together.

What makes that crucial difference is a partner's reaction to certain issues and the way compromise is dealt with. If you have this overwhelming need to feel worthy because it functions as your substitute sense of self, you may try to dominate the decision-making process. Learning to compromise can be virtually impossible for a person who's attached to a specific outcome. This can prevent your partner from doing things you disagree with, even when it's in their best interest. Without the necessary tolerance, conflicts can escalate, leading to unpleasant consequences and breakups.

If you live with someone who has a lack of sense of self, it's likely that you're playing second fiddle. When a person is dependent on realizing the conditions that are necessary for their substitute sense of self, every moment of every day is filled with trying to get there. That leaves hardly any room for genuine attention for you, as their partner.

Now is a good time to ask yourself whether this could apply to your own relationships, both past and present. Do your loved ones come second? Or are you willing to take a back seat to their wants and needs?

The scenario depicted above has similarities to the one of insomnia, in that it has the *same cause*: a lack of sense of self. This condition leads to a wide variety of symptoms, causing suffering and misfortune that affect all aspects of your life.

For years I took my inability to sleep as a sign of selfishness. All my life, my mother criticized me for having too many problems, blaming me for making *her* life miserable, as if I was doing that *to* her. When my insomnia began, her criticisms intensified. I felt inferior because of my insomnia. I was deeply ashamed of it. I was so caught up in the negative self-image that I wasn't even concerned about what was going on inside myself, how disabled I felt, or how physically unpleasant it was. What's more, it was impossible for me to get that feedback from myself because I was not aware of my authenticity, my *real* self.

Not being in touch with my real self limited my emotional range drastically. My emotions mainly swung between the fear of not sleeping and anger when I failed to fall asleep. But those feelings didn't have anything to do with my real self. The only emotions I had access to were the ones focused on achieving that feeling of worthiness and earning my substitute sense of self.

I was not present at all. Not for myself, not to my life, and also not to others (my friends, my children, my partner!). My only concern was meeting all the conditions I imposed upon myself. In retrospect, it became clear to me that I was no more than an empty shell back then.

This situation lasted for years. But once I began to look deep inside myself, I started to recognize my unhealthy patterns of thinking and behaving. With this newfound self-awareness, my sleep cycle improved.

The addictive habit of wanting to live up to all kinds of (often self-imposed) conditions works like a straitjacket that keeps you imprisoned in a toxic cycle and disturbs your nightly rest. You have to liberate yourself from this deeply ingrained tendency. Take the time to look at *the why* of your daily activities so you can heal your motivation. Focus on doing things that aren't attached to your hidden goal.

Implementing this change in yourself will help you develop a healthy sense of self.

It's crucial to *admit and accept* that there's a hidden goal influencing your motivation. The next step is to find out what your hidden goal is all about. Are you still trying to prove to your parents/caregivers that you're worth their attention? Do you still crave the love and appreciation they withheld from you during childhood? There's nothing wrong with wanting to get validation from other people as long as it doesn't affect you on an existential level. Most of us prefer to be on good terms with other people and know that we're valued. But with a lack of sense of self, you depend on getting validation to feel like you're allowed to exist, and that's an unhealthy, crippling condition.

In the end, we all need to learn to rely on ourselves. Even when surrounded by family and friends, we need to be aware that we are utterly alone in our minds and bodies. Friends come and go, and even the most intimate relationship can turn around and leave you on your own. You need to be able to live with yourself and be alone with yourself. Only then can you choose to have a companion who doesn't serve a codependent purpose. Only then can you be with someone for healthy reasons.

Imagine a society in which each individual has a healthy sense of self and no one is emotionally dependent on anybody else. This is the required setup for people to function interdependently, balancing strengths and weaknesses, completing each other, and working together toward a better life and a better world.

Unfortunately, we don't live in that world. Too many of us were never encouraged to develop a healthy sense of self, and we've become dependent on the validation of others.

By being dependent on approval, you give others the power to determine how you feel about yourself.

When others withhold their approval from you, it may be because you did something wrong. It may also have nothing to do with you. Before taking things personally, be aware that other people's actions and behaviors are based on their own motivation. And maybe these motivations are rooted in their dependency on gaining a substitute sense of self, which will cause them to overlook you entirely.

In this regard, parental mirroring is no exception. The verbal and nonverbal messages you picked up from your parents/caregivers form the foundation of your self-image. It's only natural for a child to assume that the adults in their lives speak the truth. And if you thought that your parents believed you were an annoying child, a nuisance, or a self-centered brat, the reality may have been that you were a hindrance to their ability to fulfill their own hidden agendas. Let's face it: if they were dependent on achieving and maintaining their substitute sense of self, you were set up to follow in their footsteps from the start. Whether intentional or not, when you receive the same message over and over again as a child, it gets imprinted on your mind and heart.

In my case, my husband has done his very best to help me refute my negative self-image. But he has also come to realize that this is an impossible task for an outsider, even someone highly motivated to help. Once you feel that everything about you is wrong, the only person who can change that limiting belief is you. Fortunately, when you succeed in restoring your sense of self, your sleeping problems will disappear along with many, if not all, of your other pains and discomforts.

On your path to healing your sleeping problem, it's important to identify what role your parents, teachers, and other caregivers played in the mirroring process. Growing up, were you confronted with an adequate mirror or with a distorted one?

> Adequate mirroring leads to a healthy sense of self; distorted mirroring leads to unhealthy motivation, which can lead to insomnia.

So now it's a matter of finding out how healthy your motivation is by applying the *Motivation Check*. For this exercise to be effective, you have to be totally honest with yourself. Is it possible that you're pursuing a hidden goal that impacts your ability to get a good night's sleep? If you find that your motivation isn't as healthy as it should be, then it's time to take your first steps in gaining insight into what you're really after.

To this purpose, you have to figure out what forced you to take on these unhealthy strategies during your childhood. Then you have to actively and consciously dismantle what's been causing you so much suffering: your *hidden goal*. Recognize that your hidden goal no longer serves you in your current life situation. Let the heartfelt inner knowing that you truly exist as yourself emerge within you. Thoroughly believe that you have the right to be who you already are. Then decide from the bottom of your heart that *you are your own goal* from now on. The moment you make that gigantic shift, your ultimate and overt goal will be your personal well-being and what you want to make of your life.

You can get started with this work right away by going back to that first reflective activity from Chapter 1. Only now, with all that you've learned so far, dive deeper into your questions and answers. Take a few minutes to stand in front of that big mirror and look yourself deep in the eyes. Be brutally honest with yourself as you answer these questions: *How do I feel about my insomnia? Why? Where do those feelings come from? What am I doing? What do I hope to gain? What am I trying to prove? Who am I doing all of this for? What is my life all about? What do I want my life to be about in the future?* When answering these questions, take into account that you only have one life, so make sure it's yours!

Living without some form of a sense of self is impossible. It's comparable to living without a psychological and emotional spine. Unhealthy motivation is driven by the hidden goal that compensates for a lack of sense of self.

Be careful that you don't use your life to pursue something you're unaware of. It's your life! Wake up and turn off your autopilot. Stop wasting your precious time and vitality chasing a dream you can't achieve. Throw away any unhealthy hidden goals and dedicate yourself to fully living life your way.

Identify your personal needs and direct your energy accordingly. Develop your own talents. Be your very own person! Be your own best friend and respect first and foremost your own personhood.

In Chapter 6, you'll find out how your hidden goal affects your quality of life.

SUMMARY

1. Parental mirroring begins immediately after birth. Without being aware of it, a caregiver emits verbal and nonverbal messages about their child, which

are picked up and internalized by the child. These messages reveal the parents' state of mind, their emotional involvement, and what their child means to them.

2. How a parent mirrors their child is influenced by their own childhood experiences and whether or not they have a healthy sense of self.

3. In the course of daily life, parents can unintentionally overlook their child's need for validation.

4. Adequate mirroring leads to a healthy sense of self. Distorted mirroring leads to unhealthy motivation, which can lead to insomnia.

5. The childhood strategy of seeking approval when feeling unacknowledged leads to behavioral changes that are not in alignment with the child's nature. Earning approval can become the child's main focus.

6. Being dependent on approval for your (artificial) self-experience makes you worry about how to function optimally, which can lead to insomnia.

7. Learning to compromise can be virtually impossible for a person who is attached to achieving specific outcomes.

8. By being dependent on approval, you give others the power to determine how you feel about yourself.

CHAPTER 6

How Hidden Goals Affect Your Quality of Life

Become your own goal!

As we all know by now, the inability to sleep influences all areas of life, even the most mundane. I'm not only referring to the easy-to-understand lack of energy and debilitating fatigue. Insomnia diminishes our overall quality of life through the decisions we make and the experiences we have. This sleeping problem and the underlying reason for it, a lack of sense of self, manifest in other ways too.

For example, how does your insomnia affect your love life? If you never know whether or not you'll be able to sleep, you often create an extended ritual around going to bed that you're anxious to hold on to. A lack of sleep leads to having less energy, and that can seriously decrease your libido.[1,2] If you haven't slept well, you're not likely to think, *Yeah, let's make love,* in the middle of the night or early in the morning. Desire for physical contact could also be reduced because of the anxiety surrounding your sleep. This can dampen your partner's interest in sex, too, when they place more value on your need for sleep than on their need for intimacy.

Insomnia not only has an enormous impact on your personal relationships but can also affect the lives of strangers. If you're driving while sleep deprived, your responsiveness is delayed because you have a foggy brain and you might nod off, so the risk of getting in a car accident is greater. Moreover, the risk of minor accidents, injuries, and illnesses is increased too.[3] Your resistance is lower, your muscle tension is higher, and your senses are dulled.

On top of those everyday worries and stresses, you also have to deal with all the "good" advice from other people, whether or not you ask for it. Everybody seems to know what you should and shouldn't do. "Above all, relax," is common advice. "But don't forget to be physically active every day! Otherwise, you're not really tired when you go to bed." In the search for a good night's sleep, you can find different suggestions for nearly everything you do. Some things might actually work for you, but it can also be easy to turn new attempts at self-care into vehicles for gaining approval.[4]

You might try out different diets that will supposedly help you sleep better, removing specific foods or drinks from your daily menu because someone mentioned they might keep you awake at night—all those delicious things like garlic, peppers, coffee, or red wine. If giving up a food or drink item helps you sleep better and you feel it's worth the sacrifice, that's great; if not, then don't deny yourself simply because someone else says you should. Despite your individual musical tastes, you might listen to meditation or sleep music at night. There's nothing wrong with that if you actually like it and you aren't solely driven by your insomnia. Meditation and yoga are great techniques to find inner peace, which can benefit your sleep, but they might not be for everyone. It's important to remember that whatever you do to support your sleep is done because you like it or because it enhances your quality of life.

Motivation is the key element, and it's not always what it seems. Ask yourself, *Does the idea of getting rid of my insomnia excite me? Does it give me butterflies in my stomach?* Then watch out! The subconscious urge to score approval might still be underneath your desire for better sleep without your ever being aware of it.

Isn't it ironic that your attempts to fall asleep could be serving your hidden goal? Do you see the knot that's being created in your life when you focus on getting rid of your insomnia instead of focusing on healing the issues that cause it? What you really need is to release, repel, and eliminate your hidden goal and the idea of your dependence on a substitute sense of self. All the more reason to gain insight into exactly what it is that you're chasing after.

The hidden goal that used to keep me awake at night was based on my perceived need to prove that I had value and that I was good enough to be part of a group or community. Virtually everything I did was in service of this goal: striving to be an excellent musician, to be a caring mother, and to quarrel less with my children.

These all seemed very noble on the surface; however, there was also an underlying unhealthy motivation that I was not aware of. Deeply hidden in my subconscious, I had a desire to score imaginary points toward approval by showing off. I thought that if I could do enough to earn the admiration of others, they would accept me and let me feel included. I didn't work hard to succeed in my career only for my love of music. I didn't do things only for my children's benefit or to create a better atmosphere in my home. No, I did it all hoping that others would see how good I was or how I could do everything better than they could.

One of my first Mother's Day celebrations was overshadowed by the negative feelings this goal created in me. It should have been a purely joyous occasion. It took place at a very romantic farm in the south of Portugal. I distinctly remember my daughters gifting me with a cup and a plate made of traditional Portuguese pottery. I also remember feeling guilty—and not only because I hadn't been able to sleep the night before. It was in those moments that I felt particularly bad about myself for having so much trouble with being in touch with my emotions. I sought refuge in pretending that I was happy, but I knew it was only an act. The sensation of detachment and not being able to be sincere was, in addition to not sleeping, one of the biggest pain points of my addiction to a substitute sense of self.

My lack of sense of self devastated my quality of life. My feelings of guilt and insincerity were often accompanied by anxiety when major events came up that provided me with the opportunity to score a lot of approval. Like other mothers, I used to look forward to my daughters' birthdays when they were little. I would buy balloons, a fancy cake, and presents, and my daughters and I would make invitations for the neighborhood children to come and play. But, of course, things never turned out exactly as planned. On the night before each of these celebrations, I could never sleep. Grieving my lack of energy and the inability to be cheerful, I would drag myself out of bed to face the day. Instead of giving my full attention to my child and enjoying the party, I had to pretend to be happy and hope no one would notice how tired I was. The underlying stress of the situation was obvious, but little did I realize that I was subconsciously using the event to earn feelings of worthiness.

At that time, I wasn't aware that *being cheerful* was one of the tasks I had imposed on myself to prove that I was "normal." "You always have some problem. You're never just happy. You're never just normal," were the complaints I'd heard all too often from my mother, the person whose approval I needed so badly. Without being aware of it, I had given myself the assignment of proving that I had everything under control. I needed to be the perfect mother and hostess and still find it all fun. In short, at the end of the party, I should have been able to say, "The day was a total success. I feel proud of myself." A typical case of unhealthy motivation. But I didn't deliberately choose to use my daughters' birthdays for my own unhealthy reasons! Experiencing things this way was a direct result of my dependency on approval.

No event was too big or too small to avoid the effect of my hidden goal: Sometimes I would enthusiastically set up dates with people to visit them or go do something fun together. In the moment, taking the initiative to make those plans seemed to be soundly motivated. But as the date approached, I would have terrible nights with little to no sleep, which often led to my breaking the plans at the last minute. After a while, I completely stopped considering get-togethers with other people. I knew that if I forced myself to go, I would have to fake my way through a day full of pain and suffering when it should have been fun—and only because everything I did was contaminated by that subconscious desire to score.

Life is not meant to be lived like that. Things need to be done for the right reason. Otherwise you're just concerned with living up to (self-imposed) conditions, with the unhealthy goal of making yourself feel like a real person. If you want to sleep better, it is of the utmost importance that you recognize your urge to score for approval. Investigate why you do what you do, and if an activity isn't being done for the right reason, you have to dig deeper. Only when you become aware that you're chasing after a hidden goal can you replace it by becoming your own goal. Only then are you truly living your own life. That is when your insomnia will end.

This isn't something that will happen overnight, though. Even after I had begun reconditioning myself, my old habit of scoring points for approval would find its way back into the driver's seat. Without being aware of it, my anticipation of having a fun day was turned into a vehicle for gaining a substitute sense of self. That pattern clearly existed in me while I was going through the process of restoring my sense of self. The new habit of doing things for myself was quickly overwritten in those early days, and my old survival strategy would take over again. But I eventually learned that relapse is inevitable when reprogramming yourself, and backsliding is merely a stumbling block that needs to be overcome from time to time.

I'm sharing this because it's not unlikely that you'll also experience the same issues I did. The key to dealing with these setbacks is tenacity! Over time, you'll learn to trust yourself and your instincts as you progress toward feeling safe in responding to things as your authentic self.

No matter what stage you're at in your healing process, there might be situations that will always trigger your insomnia. Later in life, when I would visit my elderly mother and stay with her overnight, I was almost never able to sleep. I would pretend to be well rested in the morning to avoid her criticism, but she wasn't easily fooled. Every time she took note of my tired face, it felt like I'd personally insulted her. I can still feel the way she would look at me, as if I'd intentionally wanted to make her suffer. "Why are you doing this to me? Why do you always make me miserable with your never-ending problems?" was the message I knew all too well. I'd learned the best way to deal with that situation: after a sleepless night, I would hurry out of bed as early as possible and quickly set the table for breakfast, just to indicate that everything was fine. But, in reality, nothing was fine; it was all theater.

When the cleaning lady was scheduled to come early in the morning, my mother was as strict as a general with me, never realizing that I wasn't a child she could order around anymore (I was in my late fifties by then). I had to make sure to be out of bed at 8:00 a.m. sharp and immediately make my bed, at the risk of her utter rejection. It was a weekly recipe for sleeplessness.

If you're dependent on approval for your feeling of self-worth, it's not surprising that you're stressed out about how you perform. Life has a way of messing up the best-laid plans; when you want something to go a certain way, it always seems to turn out differently. Add to that the small dramas that occur throughout the day, and it's no wonder your mind keeps you awake all night.

If you don't want your life to be one big performance, you must have the courage to face the truth about the shortcomings of the people closest to you. If they don't give you approval, it isn't necessarily your fault. Chances are that they also depend on a substitute sense of self, with all the consequences that entails. Try to remember that they're just people too.

Of course, environmental and personality factors play a unique role for each individual within the framework of this sleeping disorder. The big picture is the same, though! Regardless of personal circumstances and individual character traits, the overarching problem is a lack of sense of self. If you're busy chasing a hidden goal, you're not in charge of your own life.

Take a closer look at your own goals. You probably have plenty of good ideas about what gives your life meaning. There's nothing wrong with what you want to achieve, big or small. Just make sure you do it for the right reason. You must ensure that your sense of self-worth isn't dependent on the results of your actions. It's fine to be satisfied with what you do or to feel a little disappointed if you don't succeed. But be aware that your value as a person isn't determined by your successes and failures.

Here's an abstract exercise you can use to understand the nature of your motivation with more ease. Imagine that everything you do based on healthy motivation is green. Everything based on unhealthy motivation is red. If you're unsure of any particular activity, you can let your intuition figure it out.* As soon as you realize that a motivation is in the red,** you need to reject it and continue looking for a way to replace it with a green one. The more green motivations you encounter, the better you will sleep!

It's perhaps somewhat easier to handle your insomnia by looking at it as the sabotage of your substitute sense of self. If you're unable to sleep, simply state, "Hmm ... I'm not falling asleep. I must be subconsciously preparing myself to score approval with something tomorrow. What could that be?" Adjust that wrong motivation by shifting your awareness to the fact that your existence doesn't depend on that approval: "I am already ... I sense my body ... I feel my feet and my legs and my toes ..." Let go of your worries about the next day as you ground yourself through the mind/body awareness exercises from Chapter 2.

To get started with the following quality-of-life activity, imagine how the situations I described earlier in the chapter would have developed if I'd been aware of these techniques at the time. How would things have gone if I'd had a healthy sense of self instead? Think of some examples from your own life that would have had different outcomes if you'd had a healthy sense of self. Write down the way you think things would have gone if you'd been able to get a good night's sleep before that event. What would have

---

* It's extremely valuable to pay attention to your intuition, because it often knows more about you than your conscious mind does. Unhealthy motivation unfortunately blocks access to your intuition, which can tell you a lot about your motivation to do something.

** The nature of your motivation is often mixed. Sometimes you start something from a healthy motivation, but a red border runs across the bottom as a warning sign.

changed if you'd been fully present in that moment? In what ways would that have improved your quality of life?

It takes a lot of time to eliminate your sleeping problem, so why not become your own therapist and doctor? Finding enjoyment in everyday life and improving your relationships with the people around you are some of the best reasons to bite the bullet and start working toward solving the riddle of your insomnia. With the Sense of Self Method strategies you've been learning in your pocket, you can certainly do that.

In this chapter you got a picture of how your daily life can be influenced by a lack of sense of self. You also learned the importance of solving the problem of insomnia for healthy reasons. You can expect success by focusing on improving your own quality of life through introspection.

In the next chapter, you will find out what happens when a permanent setback makes it forever impossible for you to reach your hidden goal. I will highlight a number of moods and disorders that can occur when reaching your hidden goal is thwarted.

SUMMARY

1. Insomnia not only affects you at night; it also affects your quality of life during the day. Think of your relationship, your sex life, and a heightened risk of injuries and accidents.
2. Anticipation of a fun event can lead to a sleepless night when the event is serving your hidden goal.
3. Triggers can pull you back into your old goal of gaining approval. Take the time to think things

through and refresh your determination to live life for your own experience of it.

4. If you're busy chasing a hidden goal, you're not in charge of your own life.

5. Only when you become aware that you're chasing after a hidden goal can you replace it by becoming your own goal.

6. To improve your quality of life, ensure that your sense of self-worth isn't dependent on the results of your actions.

Insomnia

But it's really fear you want to talk about
and cannot find the words
so you jeer at yourself

you call yourself a coward
you wake at 2 a.m. thinking *failure,*
fool, unable to sleep, *unable to sleep*

buzzing away on your mattress with two pillows
and a quilt, *they call them comforters,*
which implies that comfort can be bought

and paid for, to help with the fear, the failure
your two walnut chests of drawers
snicker, the bookshelves mourn
the art on the walls pities you, the man himself beside you

asleep smelling like mushrooms and moss is a comfort
but never enough, never, the ceiling fixture lightless
velvet drapes hiding the window

traffic noise like a vicious animal
on the loose somewhere out there—
you brag to friends you won't mind death only dying

what a liar you are—
all the other fears, of rejection, of physical pain,
of losing your mind, of losing your eyes,

they are all part of *this!*
Pawprints of *this!* Hair snarls in your comb
this glowing clock the single light in the room

–Alicia Ostriker

CHAPTER 7

Insomnia and Depression

"Will I ever be able to show my worth?"

Most of us have experienced, at times, the negative impact lack of sleep has on almost every aspect of our daily life. Those sleepless hours leave us feeling weakened, unfocused, and depleted of vital energy.

Chronic insomnia is a looming shadow that negatively affects relationships, finances, health, and home life. It leaves some of us unable to control our weight: We feel hungry all the time because we have so little energy, and we're too worn out to exercise. Or we completely lose our appetite, which leaves us feeling frail and looking sickly. We're less motivated at work. Our productivity wanes as the hours drag by. Not being able to get through the day while the rest of the world is buzzing with vitality can make us feel isolated and lonely.

Maybe you feel ashamed of your insomnia and the problems it causes, just like I did. Sleeping when you should be awake and being awake when you should be sleeping makes it impossible to follow the rhythm of the average workday in our society. Is it surprising that depression is lurking when you're constantly under the spell of this problem?

In traditional medical science, insomnia is linked to depression,[1] but the question is: Which came first, depression or insomnia? Was I unable to sleep because I was depressed or did I become depressed because I couldn't sleep? Was it the chicken or the egg?

What is the underlying cause of depression?

Depression occurs when your substitute sense of self is out of reach, when you're unable to live up to your (self-imposed) conditions, or because external events that are out of your control prevent you from getting the approval you need.

Falling into depression is understandable when you become permanently and irreversibly blocked from reaching your hidden goal. The most obvious way this can happen is when crucial people disappear from your life, whether through death, abandonment, or absolute rejection and refusal to acknowledge your existence (being disowned or excommunicated). Losing a loved one is an impactful event under normal circumstances, but there's an extra dimension to that suffering if you were dependent on their approval.

Loss is an unavoidable part of life, and smaller losses can be just as devastating as the larger ones. Inner conflict brought on by life changes can lead to depression just as surely as the death of a loved one can. That includes the incredible change brought on by consciously eliminating your hidden goal (healing).

When you've devoted your whole life to your hidden goal, losing access to it can feel like losing a major part of yourself. It affects motivation and energy, as well as your overall desire to participate in life. In extreme cases, there may even be times when you wonder whether it would be better to stop living altogether. Whenever you feel this way, remember that restoring your sense of self and becoming your own goal can lift you out of these feelings of depression.[*]

What does this situation have to do with insomnia?

For me, there was an undeniable connection between falling into depression and being plagued by insomnia. After I had my first baby, it was impossible for me to practice music as much as I used to. I was no longer able to give my full attention to my career. And as I mentioned earlier, performing music was a vehicle I used to prove that I had value, that I was worthy of being seen and heard. My goal was to become so good at it that my parents would be proud of me.

Adding to the usual complexities of new motherhood, my baby girl was born two and a half months early. We were lucky she survived with no apparent health issues after her premature birth. By the time the dust settled, I had to go back to work, and that's where my internal challenges started. I was constantly conflicted about what I should be paying attention to. My feelings of worthiness

---

[*] If you're having suicidal thoughts, please reach out for help right away.

were dependent on both the success of my music career and on my baby's well-being.

I used to be ashamed of this lack of heartfelt devotion to my child, but I refuse to feel that way anymore. I didn't know any better. I now understand that my inner conflict back then wasn't caused by my inability to manage both taking care of my child and doing my job properly. If I'd had a healthy sense of self, I should have been able to do that. No doubt it still would have been difficult—it's sort of an unnatural situation forced upon us by the modern way of living—but many people successfully juggle family and professional functions. My problem arose because I (unknowingly) used my activities to earn a substitute sense of self.

My subconscious commitment to making things work out in ways that guaranteed my ability to feel worthy was in jeopardy. My hidden goal could no longer be my central focus. That was the moment my acute problems with insomnia showed up. I would lie awake for two to three nights in a row, and then I would be so exhausted that I would finally sleep the next one.

I wasn't really worried about my baby's well-being because I was subconsciously agonizing over very different things. Becoming a mother didn't mean that I suddenly was no longer my mother's child. And I still needed her approval more than anything. That also applied to the way I was raising my own child, so I couldn't afford to fall short. To avoid the risk of my mother's disapproval and rejection, I needed to be her interpretation of an ideal mother: An ideal mother is selfless and only thinks of her child. Motherhood makes her so happy that it overrides all her own issues. And of course an ideal mother is able to sleep so she can be well rested and fully present for her child during the day.

The combination of my role as a new mother and the ongoing pursuit of my hidden goal left me feeling paralyzed. There was no way I could do things perfectly, which provoked a lot of anxiety. Part of me wanted to work hard at getting my music career back on track so I could continue using it to score points with my mother. The other part of me wanted to be the calm, loving mother who had no trouble managing all the domestic responsibilities that come with parenthood. But above all else, I still wanted to feel worthy, and the paths leading there sent me in opposite directions. It was a no-win situation.

The quest for my substitute sense of self was falling apart, and it felt like a death sentence. Not so much physically, of course, but psychologically. The challenges were imperceptible, so I had no idea what was going on. At my wits' end, I often wondered what was driving me mad: "I am not an angry person at heart! I'm not quick to yell or lose my temper. I know I'm a fun-loving, positive person. So why do I behave like this now that I'm a new mother?"

All through the night I'd toss and turn, and then drag myself out of bed in the morning, feeling more dead than alive. I felt like I was failing on all levels: With my baby, who needed me. With my partner, who had to go to work and often acted as a substitute mother when he was home. With my mother, because I couldn't live up to her expectations of being a "normal" mother without any problems. And with myself and my intention to do right by my daughter. It felt like everything was going down the drain.

Despite all this, I still went to work every day and did my job as best I could. Even though I had very little energy,

I tried to be positive toward my baby because she was, of course, the sweetest baby in the world. From my own childhood experience, I understood how important it was to be positive with my child. But as a person, I was completely broken, and I didn't understand the reason behind it. This situation resulted in a depression that manifested as insomnia.

I was constantly angry. When something went wrong, I felt a fire ignite in the pit of my stomach. When something got in my way or if I failed to get a certain result, I would blow up. I was aware that I couldn't keep my anger contained. Even if I managed to do so for a little while, it would seep out in an unexpected moment anyway. As an attempt to lessen this at home, I crafted a stop sign out of cardboard together with my children. I told them, "When Mommy is angry again, please tell me, 'Mommy, the stop sign is red!'" I hoped they could understand that I wanted to do the right thing, but it was too hard sometimes. I couldn't sleep, and it was impossible for me to behave the way I knew I should.

My anger was a form of self-justification. It also served as an excuse. My outbursts revealed my fear of what would happen if I failed to act or behave the way I thought I should. But that fear had nothing to do with my children, my work, my mother, or my husband. *What I feared had nothing to do with reality.* The dread that my hidden goal was in jeopardy generated that fear. The belief that I had no choice but to meet all the conditions required to accomplish that goal was at the root of my fear and anger. If only I had been able to think independently and look at myself, I would have seen that I was angry because I was terrified that I wouldn't be able to get it all done.

Without feelings of worthiness, I felt like I didn't count. I was that empty shell. I had no sense of who I was. I didn't have that inner knowing that I owned the right to be myself simply because I already existed in flesh and blood. This continuous imaginary battle against some sort of metaphysical death (annihilation, rejection) is the burden of someone with a lack of sense of self.

My family and I moved abroad twice while I was going through this. First to Portugal, and then to the United States. It took about five years before I sat down at my desk for the first time and thought, *If I want to help myself and get rid of my insomnia, I have to step up and do the work myself.* During the days that separated my sleepless nights, my life was a battlefield. I wanted to continue working as a musician, so I always ran out of time at the end of the day to work out the ideas I came up with. What I didn't know then was that this new endeavor to get rid of my sleeping problem was still in the service of feeling worthy; I still did what I did for unhealthy motivation. It was much later that my motivation to truly heal myself of insomnia became for the sake of being a whole and healthy person.

Perhaps your mind is tired from not having slept well as you're reading this story and your gaze is hazy from exhaustion. Maybe you, too, are angry with your circumstances or you feel completely subjected by them. It's possible that you've lost interest in your life because there's a voice inside, telling you, *Don't bother; it won't work out anyway because I can't sleep.* Perhaps you're overcome by feelings of depression. I want you to have one thing clear: *depression has nothing to do with your real life, with your real self.* Depression comes from not being able to realize your hidden goal and gain your substitute sense of self.

What you need to do now is discover your hidden goal. If you catch yourself thinking, *Well, I don't have a hidden goal,* take a deeper look within. It can be hard to recognize because it's something you have unknowingly been carrying with you throughout your entire life. You're so used to its presence that you can't see it. *But you must find that goal and dismantle it.*

After having wholeheartedly decided that you no longer want to be the slave of what used to be your hidden goal, you then have to decide that YOU will be your own goal from now on. You now must make sure your life is really about you, and not about getting someone else's approval or keeping someone else happy, even if that person is close to you, even if that person is someone from your own family! I would like to add, *especially someone from your own family!* It's most often your parents or a close caregiver who you so desperately want acknowledgment from. Figure out whose approval you think you need and consciously stop trying to please them.

Voluntarily surrendering your hidden goal may be easier to process than having it taken from you, but it's still a huge change. You may feel like giving up on the process because it's easier to return to the way you used to do things than it is to push forward. That's a natural impulse when you let go of what used to be your strongest motivation in life. Know that you have to pass through the pain of that loss to heal and that replacing your hidden goal is the most sensible thing you can do to free yourself from insomnia.

You must make a start with really getting to know yourself as an individual who is separate from others by taking stock of your opinions, desires, and preferences. Ask yourself the following questions (and keep in mind that no one is listening, so you don't have to worry about anyone else's opinion when you answer): *What do I want to do with my life? What do I think I can do with it? What do I think of life in general? What are my values? What are my capacities? What are my talents? What are my limitations? And how can I fill my life so I can say it's been a satisfying one?* Repeat these questions to yourself throughout this recovery process. See if your answers change as your sense of self strengthens and you become less and less reliant on others.

This Sense of Self Method will not only rid you of your sleeping problem; it will also give you the tools to turn depression into feelings of vibrancy and a zest for life. Depression fits right into the picture of life with a lack of sense of self, unhealthy motivation, having a hidden goal, and dependency on approval. But keep in mind that it can be a part of the healing process too. Feeling sad or angry is a natural part of life. Allow yourself to feel the pain of loss and change as you push forward to a brighter future. After the pain of rebirth, you will appreciate the happier days to come all the more.

Remember, you *are* already existing. Make an effort to sense your body, to become aware of yourself, to feel that you are your own unique person inside and out. Look around you with eyes that you own and you will see an undeniable truth: you love life!

In this chapter, you have seen that the certainty of never being able to prove your value to your parents/caregivers or even to yourself can lead to depression or worse. By replacing your hidden goal and becoming your own goal, you will finally enjoy a restful sleep. Now, continue to

Chapter 8 to learn about the relationship between a lack of sense of self, a lack of self-confidence, fear, and insomnia.

SUMMARY

1. When the person whose approval you need to compensate for your lack of sense of self has become forever out of reach, you may fall into depression.
2. In traditional medical science, insomnia is linked to depression.
3. Since feelings of worthiness function as your substitute sense of self, this state of feeling worthy needs to be reached at all cost. Everything else has to yield to that priority.
4. Inner conflict about what to give priority can lead to nights during which you can't sleep at all.
5. Discover your hidden goal and find out whose validation you desperately need.
6. Replace your hidden goal by serving your true self: find out what makes you happy and gives you joy, and make your life about reaching those goals.
7. Be aware that dismantling your hidden goal may lead to depression, even when the change is self-imposed.
8. Becoming your own goal will help you resolve issues with anger, anxiety, depression, and insomnia.

CHAPTER 8

Self-Confidence, Fear, Anger, and Insomnia

What to do when you can't sleep.

D o you think you would sleep better if you had the inner conviction that you are enough and that what you do is enough too? What if you could fully love and believe in yourself and honor your fundamental nature? Well, for starters, you would rest easy and sleep soundly.

This chapter illuminates the root cause of your sleep problem that is shared by fear, anger, and a lack of self-confidence, as well as by a lack of sense of self.

If the frequency with which we use the word "I" were a trustworthy indicator of how much knowledge we have about ourselves, we wouldn't have to worry about what that word means. It's a tiny word, but we use it all the time. Unfortunately, using "I" doesn't imply that you've developed an adequate sense of everything it covers. *Who am I? What am I? How do I know that I'm myself? What is the self? How can I feel (sense) it?* If you don't have a clear image of yourself or you only have a negative self-image, how can you have self-confidence?

There's so much we think we "must" do and be in this world: have a good career, make money, be cool, look attractive, be an obedient son/daughter, be a loving parent/grandparent/sibling/grandchild, be in a romantic relationship, be a good role model, etc. But how can you be sure all of that is what's best for you? How can you have a firm belief that you exist as your own unique individual, separate from others, if you're unable to recognize and sense yourself? To that purpose, you need to restore your sense of self.

With a restored sense of self, you live life on your own terms and do what's right for you, whether or not others approve. It may turn out that your ideal life conforms to the expectations of others, in part or in whole, or maybe it doesn't. Only one thing is certain: this life is yours, and it belongs to no one but you.

Self-confidence* is rooted in a healthy (restored) sense of self. It implies knowing that you are and have the right to be your own person, that you have the right to your own opinions and preferences and can express them without hesitation. You don't have to please other people or win their approval to finally feel worthy. You can feel good about yourself simply for being who you are.

---

* Visit www.healthysenseofself.com for a free download of *The Secret to Building Self-Confidence* booklet.

Chapter 8

For many of us, however, self-confidence doesn't come naturally. When we haven't been in the position to develop a healthy sense of self during childhood, we have to work our way toward it later in life. Earlier, we discussed that sleeping problems could be traced back to unhealthy motivation, where you feel forced (for a sense of survival) to achieve certain results. By changing our core motivation, we need to learn to focus on what we truly need and want instead of on what we must do to get approval. We need to leave behind that addictive need to feel worthy and learn to be confident in the fact that we are enough already.

Have you ever considered what's going on in the rest of your life? Are things going reasonably well? Do you have a sense of stability? Do you have the job you want? Do you have friends and people you like around you? You can discover the culprit of your sleeping problem by examining what's going on in your life. Crucial information may be buried in your daily habits and the way you react to things.

My lack of self-confidence, for example, was accompanied by many fears and other unwelcome emotions. This constellation had everything to do with my dependency on fulfilling the conditions I thought I had to live up to. I needed my worthiness fix!

When, after the birth of my first daughter, my maternity leave came to an end, I was eager to get back with my colleagues and perform music. But along with this sudden onset of insomnia, I noticed I was increasingly irritable. I was ready to explode when circumstances were not serving me and when others didn't behave as I thought they should.

Being prone to having uncontrollable surges of emotion is one of the clearest symptoms of a lack of sense of self. I needed that substitute sense of self so badly, and the moment it was out of reach, it felt like I had lost the right to exist. Feeling worthy was of vital importance; at least, that's how I experienced it. And when everyone and everything seemed to oppose me—sometimes life is just that way—it provoked panic, fear, and anger.

Coincidentally, *not allowing myself to get angry* was one of the (self-imposed) conditions I forced myself to live up to. Even later in life, arguments with my mother were frequent, and she always blamed me for the fights. I needed her approval, so getting angry was taboo! The internal struggle to suppress my anger was one of the reasons I couldn't sleep. When I couldn't sleep and was upset about it, I felt a strong need to justify myself. I would talk to my husband to vent my charged emotions and get all the misery I'd experienced during the day out of my system. Often, expressing myself with colorful words helped me to finally fall asleep. In hindsight, I can see how supporting me in that way through all those years must have been quite a challenge for him.

Over time, I started to recognize several patterns in my insomnia. It showed up in four distinct ways: trouble falling asleep, trouble staying asleep through the night, waking up too early, and complete blank nights with no sleep at all. Sometimes I was so tired that I had to take an afternoon nap to catch up.

Eventually, I knew I wouldn't sleep after watching a movie, after having sex, after a good day, after a fun experience, or on or before a holiday—especially birthdays, Christmas, and Mother's Day. If I wanted to go to the gym early in the morning or if I had a fun outing planned, I would not sleep the night before.

Chapter 8

My sleeping problem considerably reduced my freedom of choice in what I could do with my life. Living with and taking care of young children already limited my whereabouts, and on top of that, I simply couldn't count on being fit enough to function on any given day. In the long run, I had to give up my orchestra job. Sustaining or rebuilding a life of my own, both professionally and socially, was just not possible.

In the beginning, when the sleeping problems started to act up, I kept myself in bed, desperately trying to sleep. But sleep is something you can't command to happen. The harder you try, the less you succeed. Especially when your sleeping partner is noisier than desired—sometimes, steady snoring can have a relaxing effect, but unexpected talking, intermittent snoring, heavy breathing, coughing, or even sudden movements were a challenge for me. And no matter how much they want to, your partner can't avoid making an occasional sound, an involuntary muscle movement, or rolling over in their sleep.

For me, however, these common bedroom scenes were doom scenarios. Every time I finally fell into a light sleep and something like that happened, I was wide awake and right back at the starting line. Panic would strike me like a thunderbolt, and I was terrified that, once again, I would not sleep at all that night. The fear would immediately drive an adrenaline rush through my body. No use even trying to fall asleep for the next two or three hours. But I would stay in bed because that's what you're supposed to do at night. It was a difficult time for both my husband and me because, ot course, he didn't want to be the source of my being panic-stricken and wide awake in the middle of the night. At the same time, he couldn't do anything about it either.

I started to reflect on what was happening, and my cellphone became my best friend. Questions, insights, and upsets, I began to record them all. Whenever I couldn't sleep, I would get up and pour my heart out on my recorder instead of lying unhappily between the sheets or waking up my husband. Letting him sleep peacefully made me feel less guilty and helped me relax. This new habit eased a lot of my stress and fear, and after my nightly recordings, I could actually catch some sleep. At the same time, I created an enormous amount of material, which led to significant conclusions later on.

What can you do to work on solving your insomnia during your nightly waking hours?

It's wise to use that time productively, in ways that help you gain insight and find a solution. There are three different goals you can pursue with your nocturnal activities: regulate your emotions that relate to the previous day's events, learn more about what is happening within you, and reassure yourself.

Recognizing patterns in your emotional response to what has happened to you during the day is the key to solving your sleeping problem. To get insight into how you experience things on a deeper level, you can ask yourself a million questions out loud and record your answers honestly. *Why am I not sleeping? What have I done this time? How did I feel about today? What was really going on? Whose approval was I after? Who or what made me feel negative about myself? Was I wrong to be concerned about it? Was my response justified?*

Dependency on approval usually involves the approval of a specific person. To get insight into what your (self-imposed) rules are, ask yourself what this special person would have expected from you. What would you intuitively do to earn their approval? If you know what that is, then ask yourself what you can do differently in this new phase of your life.

The voice recorder or video recorder on your phone is perfect for recording your answers to all these questions, but if you're uncomfortable speaking, you can write out your responses in a journal instead.

Productive Insomnia Activities List

- When you're highly emotional, record your feelings and review them after you've calmed down.
- If there are too many things going on at the same time, an inner conflict is likely to arise. Talk it out on your phone or write it out in a journal to try to get some clarity on the situation.
- Once you recognize patterns in your emotions, reactions, and behaviors, give them a name using your own words. Labeling these patterns in a way that fits your life and situation will help clarify what's going on with you as you keep working with the method.
- While talking about your experiences, you can get sudden, valuable insights into why you're unable to sleep at that moment. Make a note of these insights as soon as you have them because it's easy to forget what happens in those darker hours between reality and sleep.

- Have compassion for yourself. It's not your fault that you can't sleep. You don't do it on purpose, so don't blame yourself.
- Try not to let what other people say about your insomnia affect you. Keep in mind that not everyone understands this problem, and they won't recognize that it results from what happened (or didn't happen) earlier in your life.
- Know that, in general, you probably get more sleep than you think. Try to get a sense of what the reality is and relax. There are several applications available for your cellphone that measure your nightly activity, and a device like a Fitbit can help you track your sleep.
- If you don't say anything about it, others often won't notice that you haven't slept; they're usually more concerned with themselves. Even if you feel tired or down, knowing that it will likely go unnoticed can make you feel a whole lot better.
- If someone complains that you're making life difficult for them, try not to worry about it. You aren't responsible for their feelings, and you don't need their approval!
- Above all, listen back to your recordings or read what you've journaled. Nobody knows you as well as you do. Turn your passive self-knowledge into active self-knowledge and reap the benefits. Listening to the recordings or reading your notes enables you to notice the negative patterns that contribute to your insomnia. (An interesting side effect for me was that listening to my soft-spoken, monotonous recordings helped lull me to sleep; hopefully, this activity will have the same effect for you.)

The patterns I discovered in myself all pointed to the fear of not being able to perform in ways that would yield validation, appreciation, approval, or a feeling of belonging. I was scared to death of not getting that approval and ending up with nothing to fill that empty space inside.

I call this the *fear of annihilation*.[1] It's the primary fear for a person without a sense of self because it's in direct opposition to your need to be seen and heard. You want to participate in life, to be acknowledged and included. You want to feel vibrant and alive and know that others appreciate you. All those things are perceived to be at stake if you're unable to meet the conditions you have put in place for yourself.

The fear of not being able to reach that state of feeling worthy can be compared to a general state of anxiety. What follows is an important section for people who feel anxious and have no clue why.

First, let's agree on the fact that there will always be reasons for fear in life. Some situations or events are exciting because a lot depends on how they turn out. Fear is not necessarily a bad thing, and healthy fears can be quite useful.

But if fear is experienced so deeply that it touches your sense of feeling allowed to exist, you may wonder whether the fear is based in reality. Chances are, this fear of annihilation is an illusion based on conclusions you drew as a child. No doubt these conclusions served a purpose at an earlier point in time, but they've probably outlasted their usefulness. Examine them, figure out where the fear stems from, look at how it has affected your life so far, and decide that NOW is a different time—if this fear doesn't serve you any longer, it harms you.

Based on the fear of not being able to gain your substitute sense of self, you can also experience *fear of your own emotions*. This means you dread emotions that interfere with your hidden agenda, so you become afraid of experiencing things that evoke feelings you believe are unacceptable or off-limits for you. For example, suppose the person whose approval you need continuously reproaches you for being too sensitive. To refute that judgment, you have learned to monitor your emotions and go to great lengths to avoid situations and conversation topics that may upset you. Or suppose they disapprove of you when you're upset. Knowing that anger is a deal breaker for getting approval, you learn to control your behaviors and reactions so you don't appear angry.

The *fear of your own behavior* is closely linked to the fear of your own emotions because you want to keep your behavior under control for all the same reasons. This leads to compulsive micromanagement of your environment, which results in the people you live with being forced to walk on eggshells when you insist on having things just so. Of course, it also influences your situation at work as well as your relationships with friends. No matter where you are or who you're with, when you have a lack of sense of self, you need people to behave in ways that don't provoke unwanted emotions to help ensure that *you* keep that state of feeling worthy.

Living up to all kind of rules and conditions requires you to function properly, creating the fear of *not being able to function*. Anything that interferes with your ability to function—like not sleeping—scares you to death. One thing that keeps you awake, ironically, is the fear of not being able to sleep. This fear puts a lot of pressure on your ability to sleep, which is almost a guarantee for keeping you up at night.

The *fear of change* might be a more common sentiment, but if you lack a sense of self, dealing with change is especially hard. There are so many moments of change in our lives, both good and bad, anticipated or unexpected: starting a new job, new people coming into your life, marriage, divorce, moving to a new home, illness or injury, the loss of a loved one, etc. Just when you think you have your life organized the way you can handle it, the prospect of change can fill your thoughts with doom scenarios.

The *fear of failure* can contaminate any activity that requires the support of your real self. You feel like you're not standing on solid ground, not because you're incapable of doing something, but because you aren't present to yourself.

An important aspect of this fear of failure is the unhealthy motivation to prove that you have value. Events that include an audience can be acutely charged with the fear of failure when your substitute sense of self depends on the quality of your performance.

During the years I worked as a musician, I perceived so much to be at stake, so I would over-prepare for my concerts. But whenever it was time to play my solo, things usually went like this: I would make a good start, but halfway through it seemed as if I'd stepped out of my body to watch myself. While playing my piece, a teasing voice would pipe up in my head, saying things like, *What if you're off a measure? What if your instrument malfunctioned now?* The lack of a sturdy connection with my true self, together with the dependency on the outcome of my performance, caught me in this web of self-sabotaging scenarios. Needless to say that these interferences scattered my focus and ruined, if not my performance due to my almost inhuman concentration, the joy of doing it.

For years, I had nightmares about forgetting that I had a concert scheduled. In a sudden panic, when it was already way too late, I would remember, "Oh, no! I have a concert starting in five minutes! Where's my bassoon? Did I take it home or leave it in the studio? I'll never make it in time." Or I'd dream that I was at the concert location, but didn't bring the appropriate black clothes. Another horrible dream was about my reed—an essential part of a bassoon: I would be sitting on stage, ready to begin the performance, when I would see that my reed was bent or broken.

These types of nightmares and worries indicate the fear of failure. When you're doing things for healthy reasons, it's normal to experience some tension and a bit of stress. It can even work in your favor because it helps you focus on the task at hand. But if you're using things to generate feelings of worthiness, it's a different story. The problem is that the difference is not visible to outsiders; sometimes it's not even visible to you if you don't learn to differentiate between stress that is helpful and anxieties that limit your potential.

As a special assignment for this chapter, I want you to undertake something today that won't lead to approval, something that may not be met with any response or may even cause disapproval. It has to be something you want to do *for yourself*, something you've always wanted to try but were too afraid that other people might find it awkward or weird, or something your parent/caregiver would not approve of. Do it anyway, and see how much fear and tension that stirs up within you. See how much you enjoy doing it and how you feel afterward. It can also be an amusing way to examine your own tastes and desires and start to free yourself from the addiction to approval.

Once you liberate yourself from needing approval, you'll no longer worry about avoiding unwanted feelings or criticism. Owning your natural right to exist as yourself and anchoring that feeling in your heart and soul will give you the peace of mind you need to have confidence in your abilities and ultimately sleep better.

In Chapter 9, I'll introduce two elements that play an important role in the addiction to approval: the internalized parental voice (IPV) and the autopilot.

SUMMARY

1. Many of our fears that keep us awake at night are a result of trying to live up to someone else's expectations.
2. Self-confidence is rooted in a healthy (restored) sense of self. It implies being rooted in your real self without holding back.
3. Insomnia and a lack of self-confidence are both caused by a lack of sense of self.
4. Anger and rage are rooted in the fear of not being able to earn feelings of worthiness.
5. When you can't sleep, use your time to record your thoughts and feelings on your phone or write them in a journal. Collecting information about yourself can lead to insight and positive change.

6. Sleeping problems have an isolating effect.

7. A few fears that can arise because of dependency on approval are general anxiety, fear of your own emotions, fear of your own behavior, fear of not being able to function, fear of change, and fear of failure.

8. You have a natural right to exist as yourself. Once you believe it, fears will fall away and you'll experience clarity and peace of mind.

CHAPTER 9

The Nagging Inner Voice and Your Habit of Listening to It

Relapse goes hand in hand with recovery.

Your parents' reality at the time you were born isn't within your conscious awareness, but what they thought and felt about your arrival in their lives remains with you on a subconscious level. As you were growing up, their spoken and unspoken messages stuck with you, and they may still play an active role in your life, determining many of your decisions.

These messages ring through to you by means of your *internalized parental voice* (IPV), which still reverberates long after childhood. If your parents didn't have a healthy sense of self, fulfilling their own conditions came first. They may have wanted to be the best parents, but chances are they were still governed by their own IPVs and ended up passing many of the unhealthy messages they received as children on to you. This is how a lack of sense of self can be handed down from generation to generation.

In this chapter, I'll show you how your IPV, together with your autopilot, plays an important role in finding the solution to your sleeping problem.

I want to clarify that the IPV is not an actual voice in your head but rather a collection of messages about yourself and the world around you that you received as a child.[1] You may *think* that you're the one generating these ideas and beliefs, but you're just the recipient. In reality, they stem from the time you believed everything your parents taught you as well as the subliminal messages they conveyed to you. These messages grew up with you, and because you never questioned them, they're continually reconfirmed. Eventually, they become ingrained feelings and beliefs, especially the ones that are about yourself.

You may wonder how it's possible that you still accept your parents' opinions and conclusions about who you are long after childhood is over. How would you not ask yourself whether or not you agree with the way they view you and simply take their point of view as your own? Aren't these judgments rooted in the past and not reflective of the truth about you? This phenomenon is possible because, in general, people tend to function largely on *autopilot*.

Running on autopilot is going through life without actively asking yourself whether you, as your own person with your own criteria, stand behind the points of view that come up in your mind, the actions you take, and the decisions you make.

The IPV and the autopilot are mechanisms that constantly pull you back into your old patterns of behavior. They're ultimately responsible for your sleeping problem. And unless you do something to stop them from dominating you, your insomnia will continue.

Essentially, your IPV and your autopilot are intertwined, and sometimes they merge. For a deeper understanding, it's better to think of them as two separate phenomena. To free yourself from both your IPV and your autopilot, you have to get a clear idea of how these processes can keep you captive. Let's start with the autopilot.

To take back the steering wheel from your autopilot, you must first become aware that it's hidden in the depths of your subconscious. The moment it takes over, it puts you (your real self) in the back seat. That means you stay passive while it drives you. You need to become aware of this passivity and learn to recognize it so you can step up and become actively involved in the decisions you make. Even if you understand how this works, it's still challenging to intercept your autopilot at the crucial moment and shift to consciously processing your choices.

It's vitally important that you do so, though, especially when you're taken over by negative, self-critical thoughts and feelings. You can't fully live in the present when your autopilot is making decisions for you based on past conclusions.

Humans are creatures of habit, and we all live on autopilot to some extent—we wouldn't be able to function if we had to question all our actions all the time. But being dependent on approval makes it imperative to take a closer look at certain automatic thoughts, judgments, and actions, and ask yourself, *What do I truly think?*

Here's part of my morning routine as an example. Before I go to work in the morning, I always make my bed and wash my breakfast dishes. I perform these tasks on autopilot. They're practical activities, but I never wonder whether they're absolutely necessary. In fact, at some point in my life, their urgency felt so compelling that I would rather be late than leave these tasks undone. In hindsight, it would have been way better if I'd asked myself why this habit was so important to me. I would have gotten a surprising answer, revealing my true motivation.

You see, I used to be late a lot. I had that issue for most of my life, and I wanted to be able to manage my time more efficiently. So, I actively asked myself what could be behind that. Why did I always end up losing those precious minutes doing things that were irrelevant to my plans for the day? What I found had everything to do with my dependency on approval: I was doing things that I anticipated would need to be done when I returned home so I wouldn't be bothered by them then. That way I could get straight back to work on what was most important to me. In short, I wanted to free up time so I could use it to score. I wanted to use my time fully for working on building up my feelings of worthiness. I had to dismantle the messages that were fueling my autopilot to discover that disconcerting truth about my actions, and then I had to retrain myself to no longer honor those anticipatory behaviors that caused me to be late. I was able to change my behavior, but it was a slow process, and I went through a decent amount of trial and error.

Changing an ingrained behavior is harder than you think, but all it really requires is persistence. Try it out with an everyday object, something that's been sitting in the same place for years, like a clock or a trash can, and put it in a different spot. It takes much longer than you would think before you stop looking at that spot where the clock used to hang or before you stop walking up to the place where that trash can used to sit.

Making this kind of adjustment is infinitely more difficult when you're changing an intangible habit that's not easy to identify. But it's still possible.

Your autopilot plays a crucial role in your sleeping problem because it keeps the internalized voice of your parents/caregivers alive; it allows your IPV to continuously reinforce its expectations and conditions for approval.

> When you live on autopilot, you're not present enough to yourself to question your IPV, and its messages are accepted without any objection.

Your IPV can be a major obstacle on the road to change. It works like a record that keeps playing the same old song. To some extent, this can be reassuring: it feels as if the past isn't over, which means you feel justified in honoring your old survival mechanisms. But this attitude doesn't allow you to make progress toward becoming your own person.

Here's an example of an IPV that I had to dismantle:

In my family, anything related to psychology was taboo, especially for my mother. (In those days, self-help and therapy were less common.) Presenting the image of being okay was far more important than actually being okay. I carried this belief well into my adulthood. I never told my mother I was trying to get rid of my insomnia by studying myself or that I had written a book about my findings. And to this day, I feel uncomfortable and tend to criticize myself when I spend too much time working on Healthy Sense of Self material. Even though it's currently my mission in life to help others find themselves, I'm still subconsciously driven to finish new books and projects as quickly as possible. Only then will my IPV let me know that I'm okay. Putting aside that inner parental voice is stressful, and it takes a lot of energy, but it's something I've learned to face because my work is more important to me than appeasing my IPV.

Now here's the question that needs to be asked: "What do I think of it myself?" I've noticed that the moments when I feel like I need to hurry, I'm not present enough to myself to identify my IPV and find out if I agree with what I think are my own opinions. I have to consciously relate that anxious feeling to its origin and then drop it, reminding myself that, of course, I can work as long as I want to.

> Your IPV is responsible for your negative self-image.
> Why would you not like yourself?

At least, that's how it was for me. I always thought I was a selfish person, that I exaggerated the problem of my insomnia to get attention. My mother used to let me know that I only had myself to blame for my insomnia. If only I would have behaved more normally. If only I could have been happy. If only I didn't always cause or create problems.

Do you think I would have had these negative thoughts about myself if I'd been loved unconditionally? It's likely that I would have understood much earlier what a gift life is, and I would have been overjoyed to be a part of it all.

Chapter 9

Once I started to look inward, I came to a much more positive conclusion: I am a truth seeker who values honesty as a pillar of community and family life. Gaining clarity about things is my most important tool for understanding myself and the world around me. Sometimes that leads to uncomfortable discussions, as not everybody is willing to engage with me on that level. Before, I was blind to the fact that I was entitled to make my own judgment calls. I didn't actively know that I didn't have to copy my parents' values or beliefs or their judgments about me. Discovering these values about myself and accepting them as an essential part of what makes me who I am helped to greatly reduce the negative self-image I suffered from for so long.

The IPV can be a negative influence throughout your life if you don't intercept the detrimental habit of listening to it. Otherwise, refuting or obeying the messages this voice infects you with will remain the only goal in your life.

Sometimes the IPV says, "It went well. You nailed it. You met the norm." Then the (ultimately beneficial) sabotage of my substitute sense of self would instantly come into play, destroying the feeling of worthiness I'd earned with that little success. For me, that sabotage invariably manifested as a migraine.

If I slept reasonably well, for once, a little voice in my head immediately stated, "Yeah! You did it!" It felt like a pat on the back from my IPV. But I learned that this little voice was treacherous, and it put me directly back on the wrong track: the path to scoring for approval and gaining a substitute sense of self. Migraines were one of the ways my body tried to interrupt this process.

I originally thought that to stay out of trouble, I had to stop producing that little inner voice. But stopping it isn't possible. It would have meant that I'd have to be more involved with the IPV than was good for me, which can backfire and reinforce it instead. With this inheritance from the past, the key is to counteract it instead of reacting on autopilot. I learned to be positive and confirm my presence by creating personal affirmations and saying them whenever that teasing little voice spoke up: *I am already! I don't have to feel worthy. I effectively sense that I already exist and, therefore, I don't have to prove anything. I sense my body, my eyes, my ears, and so on.* Being able to say this mantra and feel my presence within my body was my proof that I existed.

Your IPV pushes you to follow the rules of your childhood survival system.[2] It urges you to score and work toward getting validation and approval. It leads to unhealthy motivation, to being a slave to fulfilling conditions, and to being absent to your own life. The sabotage of your substitute sense of self, even though it leads to insomnia, is a remedy that nature provides to help you rediscover your own voice. It wants you to proudly step forward and state, "I have nothing to prove! Not to my parents, not to other people, and not to myself! I am who I am, and I have the right to be myself, fully and unapologetically. I don't have to do or avoid anything to gain that right!"

Now, take a moment to list the negative feelings you have about yourself. What constant criticisms have you had to endure? What parts of your life have they affected? How have they impacted your thoughts, judgments, choices, and behavior?

After you've taken some time to make that list and give it some thought, ask yourself what you actually think of those negative feelings about yourself. Try to look at them from different angles and form your own judgment, regardless of what you used to think. What is the outcome of this activity? You may be positively surprised.

Now is a good time to recap everything you've learned so far and put it all together in an overview of the SoS concepts and strategies we discussed in the previous chapters. This list of the phases of the reconditioning process will give you access to all the tools that can help you heal yourself and eliminate your insomnia. It's up to you to put them to use.

1. Understand and own that you don't feel acknowledged as a unique person.
2. Investigate the strategies you developed in early childhood that helped you get your needs met. What did you do to win approval as a replacement for real attention, appreciation, and love?
3. Recognize that instead of having a healthy feeling *of* yourself, you've become an expert in how to achieve an artificial substitute for it: earning feelings of worthiness that are *about* yourself.
4. Understand that you may have become dependent on *performing* activities and behaviors that are aimed at getting approval.
5. Understand that insomnia originates from the fear that these performances will not be successful, and you will consequently be without your substitute sense of self (empty shell).
6. Remember the details of your parents' and other people's judgments and reactions to you that encouraged specific behavior.
7. Reevaluate your strategy.

8. Identify your hidden goal.
9. Release your hidden goal by becoming your new goal.
10. Learn to recognize the symptoms of relapse.
11. Get back up and continue the recovery process.

When relapse occurs, think back to the wild garden of your mind where you had to pull out the weeds to forge a new path. Your old habits are like weeds that keep trying to grow back, and sometimes they sprout up all at once, obscuring your new path until you remove them again.

After regaining your sense of self, you can still fall into the trap of cultivating feelings of worthiness when you do something that happens to be in agreement with your IPV. And, even though you've become your own goal, it's easy to miss the moment when you accidentally take the old beaten path of unhealthy behavior that enables your autopilot to resume power. When you relapse, you mistake the messages from your IPV for your own thoughts once more, and you'll likely have some trouble picking the thread of change back up again. Be patient with yourself, and remember that changing old habits is going to take time. Relapse is just part of the process.

People with insomnia seem to be more prone to relapse at night. For me, remembering my new intentions has proven to be infinitely more difficult when lying in bed. Decisions made the previous day about implementing a new behavior are freshly stored in your short-term memory and easy to lose track of overnight. A few short hours of sleep at the beginning of the night can wipe your mind clean. It's like turning off your computer without saving the data. When you wake up in the middle of the night, you don't remember a thing about the conclusions you came to the day before, the truths you revealed to yourself, or the changes you were going to make. When that happens, your old behavior takes over and with it your worries about not being able to live up to conditions, which results in not being able to fall asleep for the remainder of the night. Unless you jot down your new ideas and intentions in a journal or record them on your phone, you will be at a loss. Otherwise, getting up and reinventing them is the only way to get back on track.

It seems justifiable to let go of things when you're getting ready for sleep, but if you want to succeed in reconditioning yourself, it's a definite no-no! Lack of continuity in developing your new program leads to relapse. You need to reinforce your reconditioning program points before bed. It seems somewhat ironic that sleep itself, which is what our quest is all about, can, to an extent, be considered a roadblock on your path to becoming a healthy sleeper. Nevertheless, sleeping is necessary, of course.

When I wake up in the middle of the night and decide that I want to remain in bed, I take an important conclusion I drew earlier in the day and turn it into a mantra. This way, I use my involuntary wakefulness to strengthen my reconditioning process and benefit from it.

> *My activities are not meant to provide me with the acknowledgment I missed out on earlier in life. I don't have to prove my value with what I do or don't do. Be real! Do something because it's necessary, or because I can help someone with it. Or just because it's fun.*

When making your own mantra, you can remind yourself of things like: "It doesn't matter if I don't sleep, because my right to exist doesn't depend on what I do tomorrow. I might not be at my best, but that's okay. I'm curing myself of being dependent on approval. I'm learning to be about myself. My existence isn't dependent on my achievements. I already exist, so I don't feel dependent on what anyone else thinks of me."

If you still can't sleep after taking some time with your self-affirming mantra, ask yourself what's so important the following day. Be utterly honest with yourself, diving deep into your reasoning and any potential fears. Is it about the activity itself, or do you have a hidden goal? Do you want to please someone? Do you want to avoid disapproval?

Now tell yourself, "There's no need to worry! A bad feeling is just as valid as a good feeling. After all, good and bad feelings alternate like good and bad weather, like rain alternates with sunshine, they're both a natural part of life. Once you've had one, you can expect the other. Whether or not something is going well doesn't determine how you should feel about yourself or how someone else should feel about you."

Introspection and questioning your autopilot give you the chance to lead your own life. Eventually, these affirmations will make a difference in your self-experience and help restore your sense of self.

Knowing exactly what takes place when you relapse puts you in the position to deal with it more effectively when it happens. (Self-)knowledge is power! Trust that things will gradually get better and relapse will occur less often. There's no other option than to be content with going one step at a time. Know that by staying true to yourself more often, you are well on your way to releasing your insomnia.

In this chapter, you've become acquainted with your IPV and your autopilot, and how they lose their influence when you restore your sense of self. Relapse is something you must contend with since the power of habit is strong. But through reconditioning and determined, consistent behavior, you can win the battle.

The final chapter provides a number of examples to show you how your quality of life improves with a healthy sense of self and healthy sleep!

SUMMARY

1. Your internalized parental voice (IPV) is a set of conditioned beliefs and expectations that were passed on to you in childhood.
2. Living on autopilot prolongs your sleeping problem.
3. You can reduce the power of your autopilot by investigating your motivation and verifying if you stand behind each action, activity, and decision that it generates.
4. To dissolve your sleeping problem, you have to question each belief and expectation that your IPV comes up with. Ask yourself, *Is this really what I think of it myself?*
5. Your IPV and your autopilot lose their control over you when you restore your sense of self and make your personal well-being your new goal.
6. Relapse is inevitable, but it gets better over time.

It's not your fault!

It's not your fault
if you're anxious to step back into the groove
of trying to make it work at all cost—
often at the cost of your Self!
Trying to make your relationship work,
your marriage, your job,
your behavior, or that change in attitude ...

It's not your fault
to be so worried that, again, it won't
work because, somehow,
you always seem to screw it up!

It's not your fault
because it's in your system, hardwired into your brain.
You were trained to NOT be about your Self,
but to be about
the person who raised you.

They were everything to you: your world and your God.
How could you, as a young child,
ever have doubted them?
So it must have been because of *you*
that it didn't work.

So you still want to show the one who raised you
that they were wrong about you;
that, in fact, you *are* worth their attention,
and yes, their true acknowledgement
of you-as-the-person-you-are.

But you're still scared that *you* are
the reason it doesn't work ...
You still hope that one day your mom,
your dad, or uncle, or teacher,
who was, and maybe still is, so significant to you,
will speak the words that will change your life:

My dear, I am so sorry.
I am so sorry that I ruined your life.
I should have stood up for you when
you were being bullied,
I should have defended you instead of meekly
agreeing with those who criticized you,
I should have been there for you and held
your hand while you were growing up.
I should have realized that you are the most
precious gift that was ever given to me.
I should have valued your lovely, unique personality
instead of trying to shape you into
what I wanted you to be.
I am so sorry because I have done you
harm. Can you please forgive me?
Rest assured that it all has changed: I see you now,
and I love you from the depths of my heart.

You are my everything!

But, unfortunately, that's not likely to happen, right?
They're unable to see it from your perspective
and, therefore, they can't say it!

They only see themselves.

So, there's no use in trying to make it work!
It's time to take that vow here and now to

STOP

Stop trying to make it work
at all cost.
At the cost of your Self.

Because it's not your fault!
It's theirs.

Antoinetta Vogels

CHAPTER 10

No More Insomnia!

Now it's me who gives meaning to my life!

I n my experience, a lack of sleep isn't as perilously bad for your overall health as some people tend to think. But the many ominous articles about the dangers of insomnia scattered across the Internet can be intimidating. Is the issue of insomnia being exploited? Are the messages about the ill effects on our overall health supposed to make us freak out so we're ready to purchase specific products? It's important for those of us who suffer from insomnia to pay close attention to the source of these messages.

For me, it's obvious that insomnia is an issue that comes from within, and that none of the potions, powders, or devices being sold as a "cure" will have the long-term effect you truly need because they can't fix what's going on in your mind and your heart. There's a link between insomnia and feeling insecure about who you are, disconnected from what you do, or unsure of what you want in life.[1]

If you're ready to solve those fundamental issues, tackle your sleep problem, and improve your quality of life, here are two questions you need to be able to answer:

- How do you eliminate your hidden goal and ensure that you don't end up with an emptiness that needs to be filled?
- What does it mean to become your own goal?

To answer the first question, it's important to recognize and accept that replacing your hidden goal is a gradual process and the end goal will be reached in stages. A new habit will form as you gradually let go of your hidden goal. Give yourself permission to go at your own pace and allow your hidden goal to be your crutch until you feel strong enough to give it up completely.

Here are a couple prompts to help you remain aware of the fact that you *are* your own person. This awareness can be your lifesaver as you transition away from unhealthy habits:

- *Focus on becoming increasingly more aware of your body.* Do the mind/body awareness exercises from Chapter 2 regularly, and use them as a grounding touchstone when you recognize the symptoms of unhealthy motivation. Honor your own physicality and all other facets that belong to you: your body, your emotions, your ideas and opinions, your state of mind, the time and place in which you live, your age, your position in society, and so on. These are all aspects that can prove to you that you truly are alive, and you don't have to do anything to earn your right to exist. They are *real*, they are yours, and they are just as valuable as those belonging to other people, especially to you!

- **Learn to think with your own mind and see with your own eyes.** Remember that your perception of the world and your life experiences are unique to you. When it comes to the question of becoming your own goal, I can tell you from experience that making this a reality is absolutely worth the effort. Becoming your own goal changes everything. And this is the part where the fun comes in. This is the moment you get to decide what your own personal tastes, preferences, opinions, and desires are. Now you know you have the right to express and realize them without worrying about pleasing anyone other than yourself. Isn't that the best? After all, there's no point in sitting out your days on autopilot. And certainly not with the additional burdens that are born from not being true to yourself. Why wouldn't you want to make *yourself* your ultimate goal? After all, you only have one life, and now you know you can make it yours!

There are a few other points to remember when curing your insomnia by restoring your sense of self:

- With every activity, keep a keen eye on what you're targeting. Be aware of your end goal. Make sure your motivation is healthy when you get started and that it stays healthy as you proceed.

- Be prepared for the possibility that you may experience feelings of sadness, depression, anger, or fear from time to time, particularly in the beginning. It's okay to allow yourself to feel these emotions. They're a normal part of life, and they serve to enhance your appreciation of the brighter days ahead of you.
- The established dominance of your IPV and autopilot make relapsing into old patterns of behavior an inevitable part of the process. Don't let it deter you when it happens! Gently move yourself back into the driver's seat of your life and keep moving forward.

You can consider yourself to be well enough informed in the Sense of Self Method to put it into practice now, but you will undoubtedly encounter situations that this book doesn't describe. Each person is different, and everyone's circumstances vary. Culture determines a big part of your (old) behavior, including both your family culture and the larger culture in which you live. Specific characteristics that belong to the period in which you grew up can also have a strong influence on how you think and what you do. Don't be discouraged by these variables or the unexpected situations that may arise. One thing almost always remains the same: it's all about how to make your life yours.

Life changes drastically when you choose to put yourself first. And contrary to how it may sound, putting yourself first actually makes you less selfish.

When you restore your sense of self, you're no longer dependent on all the conditions your substitute sense of self relies on. Your inner stress about living up to those perceived obligations is gone, and that leads to having a lot more patience. You feel calmer when faced with unexpected situations, and you can think things through before taking action. You're able to be fully present when listening to other people, and you can do things for them without the unhealthy expectation or anticipation of their approval. In fact, you can finally see other people for who they are. You no longer see others as a means to the sole end of making you feel worthy. The strange thing is that you automatically become more interested in other people and that the reverse is true as well: people, in turn, become more interested in you.

Here's an example of how major this change can be, even in minor situations. Imagine your roommate is upset because she lost her phone. "I'm expecting an important call, and I don't know what to do," she says, holding back tears. If you're (subconsciously) busy with your hidden goal, you think, *Oh, no! I don't have time for this now. I'm in the middle of doing something else.* You panic because you fear this sudden interruption might prevent you from reaching your hidden goal.

This dilemma creates a huge inner conflict because you feel a pressing need to stay focused on your current task, but you also don't want to disappoint your friend. Note that you're not even considering the situation your friend is in. You hear her talk, but you're not able to pay attention to her. You might make a halfhearted attempt to help her search, or you may make an excuse to avoid helping her at all. Either way, she'll likely notice your lack of care, and it could put a strain on your relationship.

But imagine what a good friend you could be with a healthy sense of self. If you feel secure in yourself, you're able to live in the present and give your full attention to things as they happen. In this scenario, you would understand the predicament your friend is in, take a break from whatever you're doing, and be there for her when she needs you. Not only would you genuinely want to help her, but you also wouldn't resent having to pause what you're doing and give up some of your time. Whether or not you find her phone, she'll know you're someone she can count on, and it will strengthen your friendship.

To get a view of how a healthy sense of self can have a much larger impact on your life and the lives of those around you, imagine being the parent of young children. No matter how well behaved they are, children don't make life easier. And if you need to earn your substitute sense of self, they certainly can contribute to the complexity of getting this done. As parents, we want to give our children the attention they need, but when our focus is divided between them and the drive to attain a substitute sense of self, it can mess up even the best of intentions.

If *you* are your only goal, then your children's needs will be a natural priority. You'll be able to see them as both an important part of your life and as separate individuals with lives of their own. You'll be present to their ups and downs, and you'll have the ability to really "see" them and acknowledge them for who they are. This is the setting we want them to grow up in because it provides them with resilience[2] and the foundation they need to develop their own healthy sense of self.

That healthy family constellation is a revolution in a nutshell, in the world as a whole! If you can pass along a healthy sense of self to the next generation, you are contributing to making the world a more beautiful place. How you feel and behave reverberates into the people around you, and solving your sleeping problem can have a massive butterfly effect on your environment. But above all, it's your happiness that's at stake. And one of the keys to achieving that is to avoid listening to your IPV.

Maybe you're one of the people who thinks, *I'm not worthy of love*. If you don't believe you're worthy of love, it's impossible to recognize or accept love when it's offered to you. With a lack of sense of self, you're also unable to fully give love to others because your negative self-image clouds your heart and your mind.

If you do find love, whether it's platonic or romantic, the state of your sense of self often determines how things go. If your friendship or marriage is going through a crisis, you don't immediately give up on the relationship. You know you used to love each other, and maybe you still do. But, in the course of life, problems aren't always intercepted or addressed until they eventually come to a head. If you're not well rested and don't have the right energy, your reaction to a conflict may not be what you want it to be. If you're afraid of losing or not getting your substitute sense of self, you may wind up continuously justifying yourself instead of trying to resolve the issue. With a healthy sense of self, you have the patience and the receptivity to open yourself up to the problems of the other person, discuss the issues, and hopefully come to a good solution.

If you're advancing in age and retired or getting close to retirement, you stand a better chance of having a satisfying life as a senior. Retiring is something that some of us do happily and of our own free will, but for others, it's not easy at all. Make sure that you're not dependent on your social position or your work identity for your (artificial) sense of self. It'll make it much easier to focus on enjoying life, maintain good health, and sleep well so your golden years can be a positive experience.

No matter your age, there are health concerns when it comes to stress. And the constant stress that accompanies fulfilling all the conditions attached to your hidden goal can't be ignored. Anxiety and insomnia can lower your resistance and undermine your health, making you much more susceptible to catching an infection when they're going around. With a healthy sense of self, your stress levels are lower, you're better rested, and your body has more energy to fight off bacteria and viruses.

You also have less need for any medicines or other substances that are used to help you sleep or mask that you're not comfortable in your skin. Having a healthy sense of self makes you comfortable with yourself, and you don't need anything to supplement that.

The major issue of insomnia boils down to your body just needing sleep to recharge its battery, and your mind functions better in a well-rested body. That's the only good reason for wanting to have a consistent, healthy sleeping pattern, not because there's still some part of you that wants to score! If you aren't dependent on other people's approval, if you do things because you want to do them, you won't have problems with self-sabotage. Undertaking things with healthy motivation makes you prone to being successful. And what's more, you will radiate the healthy energy that drives you. Other people sense that, and it results in attracting others who are better attuned to their own personalities and to yours.

If you are yourself, you sleep as nature intended. You become calmer, and interactions with your family, friends, and coworkers are more pleasant. Your environment seems more peaceful, and other people seem friendlier. There are plenty of reasons to take action now and start working toward the life you deserve!

In the course of this book, you've seen that insomnia is a sign that something inside you is screaming to be adjusted and that restoring your sense of self is the long-term, drug-free answer to solving that problem. Since you've become familiar with the main strategies in the Sense of Self Method and learned how to implement them, you should get started right away. This is where it gets interesting! Who are you really? What do you like? What's important to you? What would you like to direct your life's energy toward, now that you're in charge of it yourself?

I wish you lots of success on the road to discovering the answers!

CONCLUSION

Now that you've reached the final pages of this book, I encourage you to think of yourself as a person who has the same rights as everyone else, which includes self-management. Just by virtue of existing, you have the right to be your own boss and to organize your life following your personal tastes and preferences. Creating that opportunity for yourself contributes greatly to a healthy sleep pattern.

But also keep in mind that the guidelines in this book are not set in stone. You don't have to practice the SoS Method exactly as it's described here. It's not about doing things precisely as I did. Your background and circumstances are unique to you, so be flexible and bend the rules to best serve your individual needs. If you find that you need to alter some things to fit your story, that's okay! Take what works for you and change anything you need to change. The main thing is to get a clear feeling for when you're living life for your own experience of it and to take action to shift back to your real self when you're compromising your values for unhealthy purposes.

You should never give priority to your *doing* over your *being*. And, weirdly enough, *being* doesn't require a lot of effort. *Being* takes place naturally in the vibrancy of life. It's a matter of being open to assessing and accepting your place in the totality of things, allowing neither shame nor conceit to create a judgment about your existence.

Life is so big, the Universe so grand, and "I" am just a speck who is allowed to be here for a very short time. Awareness of this dimension of existence is certainly a concept I want to draw attention to as an aspect of helping you back to getting a good night's sleep. When I started to write about my findings, I was convinced I had *the* solution. I thought I could change the world, but instead, the world has changed me. To set myself up for success and be happy, I had to draw the conclusion that my self-worth doesn't depend on my ability to change the world. My *being* is not defined by my *doing*.

How does that translate for you? What is your mission in life? Make sure it's based on healthy motivation!

When I first moved to the United States, my wish of owning a vegetable garden was finally fulfilled. The soil was fertile and the plants did well. We carried bin after bin of large red tomatoes to the kitchen all through the summer and into the fall. The weather remained gentle and the crop flourished, but a severe night frost befell my beautiful tomatoes at the end of November. Struck by the sight of so many unripe fruit buried under the snow, I felt sorry for them. Those poor tomatoes were still green, and I knew they would never make it. It would be their fate to freeze to death before they could reach maturity.

That image left a deep impression on me. I felt that it could apply especially to those of us who have insomnia.

It's not your fault you grew up in an environment that was unfavorable to the development of your sense of self. But luckily, you're not like the unfortunate tomatoes that were unable to speed up their maturation or move to a warmer location. No matter your situation, you don't have to feel trapped in your past or in an unhealthy environment. It's never too late to do something about your situation. I know what it means to suffer from insomnia, year after year, without hope. I didn't accept that fate, and I hope you don't either.

So please, use this book to propel yourself forward, heal your negative self-image, and improve your quality of life. Become vibrant, like the buzzing wings of a dragonfly. Become alive, like the rustling leaves of a tree moved by a warm summer breeze. Let your joy for life unfold like ripples on the surface of a lake. Greet each new day like a cat or dog, eager to play. Find satisfaction in the beating of your heart and the pulsing of blood through your veins. Because those are the things that count. Be who *you are* deep down inside. Go and celebrate your existence! You only have one life—make sure it's yours!

APPENDIX A

Types of Insomnia

The American Psychological Association recently updated their definition of insomnia in *DSM-5*. They now define it as "a predominant complaint of dissatisfaction with sleep quantity or quality." The key features listed are significant distress and/or impaired function due to lack of sleep or poor sleep quality.[1]

Insomnia is such a common sleep disorder, the CDC reports that one-third of adults in the United States suffer from insufficient sleep.[2]

It usually appears as either onset or maintenance insomnia, but some may experience a combination of both[3]:

- *Onset* insomnia is characterized by difficulty with falling asleep at the beginning of the night.

- *Maintenance* insomnia describes difficulty with staying asleep. This can include either waking up intermittently during the night or waking up too early and being unable to fall asleep again.[4]

According to Stanford Health Care, insomnia tends to be classified by how long it lasts.[5] Here are the terms for duration they list, along with a few others defined in materials from the National Sleep Foundation, *DSM-5*, and *Psychology Today*.[6]

- *Transient* insomnia lasts less than one month.
- *Episodic* insomnia last one to three months.
- *Recurrent* insomnia is two or more occurrences of episodic insomnia within a year.
- *Short-term* insomnia lasts between one and six months.
- *Persistent* insomnia lasts longer than three months.
- *Chronic* insomnia lasts more than six months, according to Stanford Health Care. However, other sources define it as long-term insomnia that occurs three or more nights per week for three months or longer.

Insomnia can also be categorized by its cause, or lack thereof.

Many people will experience *adjustment* insomnia at some point in their lives. According to the American Sleep Association, studies show that 15 to 20 percent of all adults experience this type of insomnia at least once a year.[7] Also called *acute* or *situational* insomnia, it only lasts somewhere between a few days and a few weeks, although it does have the potential to turn into chronic insomnia. It's generally associated with stress, excitement, life events, environmental disturbance, or changes in schedule. Adjustment insomnia usually abates once the cause has been resolved or you've adjusted to the change that interrupted your sleep cycle.

Primary insomnia isn't accompanied by any other medical or psychological condition, or brought on by medicine or other substances. This also includes *idiopathic* insomnia, which has no known cause.

Secondary or *comorbid* insomnia is one of the most common types, and it occurs alongside another medical or psychiatric condition. Stanford Health Care also explains that it "does not have to be caused by or change with the coexisting disorder." However, the added presence of insomnia could make the other condition worse or harder to treat. There are a number of conditions that are highly likely to cause insomnia, according to the Mayo Clinic.[8] Mental health disorders like anxiety, depression, and post-traumatic stress disorder, as well as medical conditions like chronic pain, cancer, heart disease, overactive thyroid, and Alzheimer's disease, can cause insomnia.

The Mayo Clinic also lists a number of situational or lifestyle issues that contribute to insomnia that are related to stress, travel, work schedule, and sleep habits.

Although there are many ways to categorize insomnia, all the sources used to create this appendix agree that no matter the type or the cause, insomnia is a disruptive condition that has a huge impact on your quality of life.

APPENDIX B

Psycho-Emotional Stress Insomnia (PESI)

A specific type of chronic insomnia the guidelines in this book can heal.

Based on my personal experiences with finding a solution for my chronic sleeplessness, I have created a specific category of insomnia to give a clear indication of which type of sleep disturbances the Sense of Self (SoS) Method can solve. In this appendix, I'll discuss what psycho-emotional stress insomnia (PESI) entails.

I believe the PESI sleep disorder is caused by the psychological stress of living without a sense of self. PESI occurs when a dependency on approval develops to provide a temporary feeling of worthiness, which serves as a substitute sense of self, and earning this substitute sense of self becomes the person's life's purpose.

Due to the resulting overwhelming need for approval, a person with a lack of sense of self perceives that their life depends on fulfilling certain conditions. These conditions are mostly self-imposed but are based on their parents' and other caregivers' desires to have them behave in certain ways that enable the parents'/caregivers' best performance of their own conditions. The stress caused by this situation—plus the absence of a healthy sense of self as their virtual spine to support the person—can cause severe insomnia.

The actual actions/behaviors through which this dependency on approval manifests are different for each individual. These are based on personal circumstances: the environment in which a person is raised; the nature and preferences of their parents, teachers, and other caregivers; and a person's individual reaction to each of these circumstances.

An unlimited variety of individual backgrounds may have contributed to the previously unrecognized common link between these stressors, but the SoS Method considers the addiction to a substitute sense of self to be the universal root cause of this particular type of insomnia. Grouping the multitude of stressors that induce Psycho-Emotional Stress Insomnia under this umbrella shines a light on the cure: restoring your sense of self. Freeing yourself from the dependency on approval provides you with a lifetime of peaceful, restful sleep.

APPENDIX C

Substitute Sense of Self Sabotage

Short Definition:

The intentional (but subconscious) sabotaging of the substitute sense of self, which is gained through approval-seeking behavior that leads to a temporary feeling of worthiness. It is a natural process that helps you destroy this substitute sense of self, so your real self has the opportunity to emerge.

Long Definition:

Before diving into the details of what substitute sense of self sabotage is and what it does, let's first look at the definitions of *sabotage* and *self-sabotage*.

- *Sabotage* means to deliberately damage, destroy, undermine, or cause the failure of something (so it does not work correctly or the intended goal is not achieved). It is usually aimed at gaining a political, military, or business advantage.
- *Self-sabotage* is not officially defined in any of the leading dictionaries, but it's commonly understood to indicate that something which promised to go well is unconsciously destroyed by the person's own doing.

Where the word sabotage implies an apparent goal, this conventional meaning of self-sabotage leads to the assumption that it's an act without any purpose because there's no advantage to it. There is no point in sabotaging yourself.

So far there hasn't been any insight into the fact that many people don't live their lives based on their real self but on an artificial substitute for it. The SoS Method proposes that the *self* in self-sabotage doesn't refer to the real self but to the substitute sense of self—specifically, because your real self would never sabotage the real you or any directly motivated action. Indeed, there IS no point in it!

However, looking through the lens of the SoS Method, you can see the connection between self-sabotage and the coveted feeling of worthiness, which functions as your substitute, or artificial, sense of self. By destroying your substitute sense of self, your real self has an opportunity to surface, and that is definitely an advantage, as well as a legitimate reason for the sabotage to take place.

Substitute sense of self sabotage comes into play when you lack a sense of self. You feel invisible, and you're scared of not being seen or heard or taken into account as a real person. This creates a dependency on fulfilling conditions that give you a temporary feeling of worthiness.

Living up to these (perceived) expectations seems like a life-or-death situation because failure leads to the (fictional) sense that you don't exist as a real person. The feeling of worthiness is a substitute for your real self, giving you an artificial sense of having the right to exist. It feels good, but it's temporary, which leads to a lot of fear and anxiety around losing it. Dependency on a substitute sense of self propels you into a never-ending cycle of doing whatever you can to achieve it. It traps you in a life that's not really yours.

When you live your life chasing this feeling of worthiness, you may feel as if your own body is working against you. Just when you think you've reached the point where you can safely feel good about yourself on that existential level, it seems to generate symptoms that destroy any feelings of worthiness as quickly as they appear. Or you may find yourself subconsciously doing things to sabotage your substitute sense of self. You experience this sabotage as if it isn't *done by* you but instead *happens to* you. It almost feels like you're the victim of unseen forces.

Substitute sense of self sabotage can be subtle when it affects your normal daily activities. These upsets in your regular routine may seem minor, but they can have a significant emotional impact because they block you from gaining approval and feeling worthy. It's much easier to recognize substitute sense of self sabotage when it's attached to more significant life events. Here are some examples:

- You finally convinced your dad to go camping with you, but now you're sick.

  The questions you need to pose to yourself here are: Why were you so eager to go camping with your dad? Was it only because you thought it would be fun? Or did you have a hidden agenda? If so, what was it?

- You finally got accepted into that dance program you set your sights on, but now you're unable to sleep.

  The questions here are: Why were you so eager to join that dance program? Was it really because you love dancing? Or was there something else driving you on a subconscious level?

- You finally have more responsibility at work, but now you can't seem to focus on the task at hand and you make a lot of mistakes.

  The question here is: Did you really want that promotion for yourself or were you trying to use it to feel some kind of self-worth? Were you trying to impress someone? If so, who?

- You finally get the feeling your spouse/parent/boss really appreciates you, but now you keep doing or saying things that irritate them when trying to win their approval.

  The question here is: Why do you want their approval so badly?

Any behaviors or issues that prevent you from obtaining or maintaining the temporary feeling of worthiness you need—especially at the moment you are almost there— often are symptoms of substitute sense of self sabotage.

This is how nature steps in to either destroy or prevent you from achieving your substitute sense of self in favor of being your real self.

Substitute sense of self sabotage is the way your real self lets you know that you're being ruled by unhealthy motivation, which is preventing you from living an authentic life. When you experience substitute sense of self sabotage, you need to examine your motivation. Dig into the reasons behind your behavior and find the root cause. Then ask your real self what you genuinely want. What do you want to do or avoid?

Here is the key: substitute sense of self sabotage is a natural process. Its purpose is to help you destroy your artificial sense of self and break free of the constant, painful need to do things that make you feel worthy of being alive. It gives you the opportunity to switch gears and follow a different path, the path that leads to being your real self, so you can finally start living your life for YOU.

APPENDIX D

The Twelve Sense of Self Reconditioning Statements

The Twelve Sense of Self Reconditioning Statements are the keys to unlocking your best self and finally getting a good night's sleep.

Once you learn how to identify the nature of your motivation and gain enough insight into your early childhood experiences, you'll be ready to shake off the shackles of your addiction to approval. Put these statements to positive use so you can begin living life with more mental and emotional freedom.

    I.   My life and my body are mine.
    II.   I experience myself directly.
    III.   I am present to the Here and Now.
    IV.   I think for myself.

V.   I am consciously aware of my senses.

VI. I have access to my own feelings, preferences, and opinions.

VII. I see other people for who they are.

VIII. I have conversations to transfer information or to connect with others.

IX. My work is aimed at the obvious, direct outcome.

X.   Relapse is always lurking.

XI. I am ready to share my life with others.

XII. I am ready to be part of a healthy community.

APPENDIX E

Benefits of a Healthy Sense of Self

Below is a list of benefits the Sense of Self Method claims to help people achieve when they successfully restore their sense of self. For the purpose of clarity, I've arranged these benefits into categories based on the topics they're most aligned with.

Addiction:

- Less substance abuse
- Fewer cravings
- Less compulsion to give in to addictive behavior
- Less desire to escape reality

Aging:

- Potentially less susceptible to age-related diseases
- More feelings of fulfillment
- Less worried about/more accepting of aging appearance
- Greater enjoyment found in retirement and the golden years
- Greater desire to maintain health for improved longevity

Anxiety and despair:

- Fewer panic attacks
- Fewer rages
- Decreased depression
- No suicidal thoughts or acts
- Less erratic behavior
- Increased feelings of joy, happiness, and contentment
- Increased vitality and success
- More self-acceptance and acceptance of others

Child rearing:

- More patience
- Better parenting skills
- Fewer family upsets
- More respect for children's needs
- Improved overall well-being for the child
  - o Less distracted
  - o Increased desire to learn
  - o Better performance in school

o   Better relationships with teachers and peers
o   Less rebellion

General health and well-being:

- Better overall health
- Better sleep
- More awareness of personal health needs
- Healthier habits
- Less stress, which leads to fewer stress-related ailments
- Less eyestrain
- Fewer migraines and headaches
- Better functioning digestive system
- More relaxed nervous system
- Less prone to accidents caused by a lack of focus or awareness
- More vibrant and active

Harmful or destructive behavior:

- Fewer outbursts
- Less uncontrollable behavior (i.e. temper tantrums, meltdowns)
- Less over-reactive
- Less retaliation or desire for revenge against perceived wrongs
- Less violence
- Fewer fights and arguments
- More responsible behavior
- Less careless spending and fewer issues with money
- More in tune with common sense
- Greater awareness of surroundings

- Greater desire to be part of a healthy community
- Greater desire to be a functioning member of society

Professional success:

- Clearer understanding of talents, abilities, and limitations
- Better focus at work
- Less prone to workplace injuries
- Less vulnerable to workplace bullying
- Better relationships with coworkers and managers
- Better equipped for teamwork
- Better equipped to deal with criticism
- Better able to communicate and defend ideas
- More confident when asking for a raise/promotion
- More in tune with personal goals
- More likely to achieve goals
- Less fear of failure

Relationships:

- Better chance to find, give, and receive love
- Less controlling of others and situations
- Increased comfort around others
- Increased comfort with being alone
- Better companion
- Better social skills
- Better communication skills
- Better able to recognize healthy and unhealthy relationships
- Lower chances for divorce (in a healthy marriage)

Self-realization:

- Higher overall quality of life
- More self-confidence
- Less self-critical
- More self-accepting
- No self-sabotage
- More realistic—more real
- Better balance between head and heart; genuine and integrated feelings
- More compassion and empathy
- Less self-sacrificing
- Better able to define and defend personal boundaries
- More comfortable with self-expression
- Clearer sense of personal preferences, tastes, and opinions
- Better sense of personal desires
- Better aligned with personal "blueprint"
- More inner peace
- Able to self-realize and live life to the fullest

N O T E S

Author's Note

1   Bessel van der Kolk. *The Body Keeps the Score: Brain, Mind, and Body in the Healing of Trauma* (New York: Penguin Books, 2015).

Chapter 1

1   Portico Network. "What is Developmental Trauma / ACEs?" Accessed February 28, 2020. https://www. porticonetwork.ca/web/childhood-trauma-toolkit/ developmental-trauma/what-is-developmental-trauma
2   National Council of Juvenile and Family Court Judges. "Finding Your ACE Score." Based on CDC-Kaiser Study. October 2006. https://www.ncjfcj.org/publications/ finding-your-ace-score/
3   Guy Roth & Avi Assor. "The costs of parental pressure to express emotions: Conditional regard and autonomy support as predictors of emotion regulation and intimacy." *Journal of Adolescence* Vol. 35, 4 (January 2012): 799–808. DOI: 10.1016/j.adolescence.2011.11.005.

Chapter 2

1   Daniel P. Chapman, et al. "Adverse childhood experiences and sleep disturbances in adults." *Sleep Medicine* Vol. 12, 8 (September 2011): 773–779. DOI: 10.1016/j.sleep.2011.03.013.
2   Ece Mendi & Jale Eldeleklioğlu. "Parental Conditional Regard, Subjective Well-Being, and Self-Esteem: The Mediating Role of Perfectionism." *Psychology* Vol. 7, 10 (January 2016): 1276–1295. DOI: 10.4236/psych.2016.710130.
3   Minke M. van de Kamp, et al. "Body- and Movement-Oriented Interventions for Posttraumatic Stress Disorder: A Systematic Review and Meta-Analysis." *Journal of traumatic stress* Vol. 32, 6 (December 2019): 967–976. DOI: 10.1002/jts.22465.

Chapter 3

1   The Global Association of NLP. "Definition of NLP." Accessed February 28, 2020. https://anlp.org/knowledge-base/definition-of-nlp
2   Louise Maxfield & Roger M. Solomon. "Eye Movement Desensitization and Reprocessing (EMDR) Therapy." American Psychological Association, July 2017. https://www.apa.org/ptsd-guideline/treatments/eye-movement-reprocessing
3   Bessel van der Kolk. *The Body Keeps the Score: Brain, Mind, and Body in the Healing of Trauma*, Chapter 15, 250–264 (New York: Penguin Books, 2015).
4   Neurolink. "What is NIS?" Accessed March 23, 2020. https://www.neurolinkglobal.com/what-is-nis/

Chapter 4

1   The Sleep Council. "Perfect Sleep Environment." Accessed February 28, 2020. https://thesleepcharity.org.uk/?s=perfect+sleep+environment

2   The Better Sleep Council. "The Ideal Bedroom; Extreme Remake: Bedroom Edition." Accessed February 28, 2020. https://bettersleep.org/better-sleep/the-ideal-bedroom/

3   SleepFoundation.org. "Sleep Tips for Insomnia Sufferers." Accessed February 28, 2020. https://www.sleepfoundation.org/insomnia/symptoms/sleep-tips-insomnia-sufferers

Chapter 5

1   Jessica L. Hamilton, et al. "Childhood Trauma and Sleep Among Young Adults With a History of Depression: A Daily Diary Study." *Frontiers in Psychiatry* 9 (December 2018): 673. DOI: 10.3389/fpsyt.2018.00673.

2   Desiree W. Murray, et al. "Self-Regulation and Toxic Stress: Foundations for Understanding Self-Regulation from an Applied Developmental Perspective." OPRE Report #2015-21. US Department of Health and Human Services. February 13, 2015. https://www.acf.hhs.gov/opre/resource/self-regulation-and-toxic-stress-foundations-for-understanding-self-regulation-from-an-applied-developmental-perspective

Chapter 6

1   Jae Wook Cho & Jeanne F. Duffy. "Sleep, Sleep Disorders, and Sexual Dysfunction." *The World Journal of Men's Health* Vol. 37, 3 (September 2019): 261–275. DOI: 10.5534/wjmh.180045.

2   Juliana M. Kling, et al. "Association of Sleep Disturbance and Sexual Function in Postmenopausal Women." *Menopause* Vol. 24, 6 (June 2017): 604–612. DOI: 10.1097/ GME.0000000000000824.

3   Damien Léger, et al. "Insomnia and accidents: cross-sectional study (EQUINOX) on sleep-related home, work and car accidents in 5293 subjects with insomnia from 10 countries." *Journal of Sleep Research* Vol. 23, 2 (April 2014): 143-152. DOI: 10.1111/jsr.12104.

4   Charlotte Lieberman. "How Self-Care Became So much Work." *Harvard Business Review.* August 10, 2018. https:// hbr.org/2018/08/how-self-care-became-so-much-work

Chapter 7

1   David Nutt, et al. "Sleep disorders as core symptoms of depression." *Dialogues in Clinical Neuroscience* Vol. 10, 3 (September 2008): 329–36. https://www.ncbi.nlm.nih.gov/pmc/articles/PMC3181883

Chapter 8

1   Marvin Hurvich. "Psychic Trauma, Annihilation Anxieties And Psychodynamic Treatment. For New Orleans APA Panel 'Trauma: Obvious and Hidden: Possibilities for Treatment.'" (2006). https://www.apadivisions.org/division-39/sections/ childhood

Chapter 9

1   Pete Walker. "Emotional Neglect and Complex PTSD." Accessed February 28, 2020. http://pete-walker.com

2   Whitney Norris. "Some thoughts on thoughts: The inner critic and self-talk." *Counseling Today.*

December 6, 2018. https://ct.counseling.org/2018/12/some-thoughts-on-thoughts-the-inner-critic-and-self-talk/

Chapter 10

1   Laura Palagini, et al. "Adult Insecure Attachment Plays a Role in Hyperarousal and Emotion Dysregulation in Insomnia Disorder." *Psychiatry Research*. Vol. 262 (April 2018): 162–167. DOI: 10.1016/j.psychres.2018.01.017.
2   Ann S. Masten, et al. "Resilience in Development." *Oxford Handbook of Positive Psychology* 3rd edition, Chapter 12, 117–132 (Oxford, United Kingdom: Oxford University Press, 2009).

Appendix 1

1   Substance Abuse and Mental Health Services Administration. "Impact of the DSM-IV to DSM-5 Changes on the National Survey on Drug Use and Health: Table 3.36: DSM-IV to DSM-5 Insomnia Disorder Comparison." June 2016. https://www.ncbi.nlm.nih.gov/books/NBK519704/table/ch3.t36/
2   Centers for Disease Control and Prevention. "Sleep and Sleep Disorders." Accessed February 28, 2020. https://www.cdc.gov/sleep/index.html
3   National Sleep Foundation. "What is Insomnia?" Accessed February 28, 2020. https://www.sleepfoundation.org/insomnia/what-insomnia
4   Harvard Medical School. "Too early to get up, too late to get back to sleep." *Harvard Women's Health Watch*. Update May 1, 2018. https://www.health.harvard.edu/staying-healthy/too-early-to-get-up-too-late-to-get-back-to-sleep
5   Stanford Health Care; Stanford Medical Center. "Insomnia: Overview, Causes, and Types." Accessed February 28,

2020. https://stanfordhealthcare.org/medical-conditions/sleep/insomnia.html

6   Psychology Today. "Insomnia." February 2019. https://www.psychologytoday.com/us/conditions/insomnia

7   American Sleep Association. "Adjustment Insomnia." Accessed February 28, 2020. https://www.sleepassociation.org/sleep-disorders/insomnia/adjustment-insomnia/

8   Mayo Clinic. "Insomnia: Symptoms & Causes." Accessed February 28, 2020. https://www.mayoclinic.org/diseases-conditions/insomnia/symptoms-causes/syc-20355167

ACKNOWLEDGMENTS

The birth of this book was not an easy one. After a maybe somewhat premature birth of its Dutch equivalent, a lot of research was done to underpin the conclusions and suggested healing methods for those of us who suffer from insomnia. A heartfelt thank you to Dr. Bessel van der Kolk's invaluable book: *The Body Keeps the Score: Brain, Mind, and Body in the Healing of Trauma.*

And another heartfelt thank you to our in-house editor, Nora Smith, who felt inspired and dedicated long hours of hard work to do the background research that supports the hunches and discoveries I made in my own healing process.

The publication of this book has also dramatically benefited from Raghenie Bhawanie, my (former) teammate in the Netherlands and her loved one. Thank you for your critical thinking and your dedicated improvements, both in living Dutch as well as in content logic. Your constant attention to ensuring that readers who are new to the Sense of Self Method and have picked up the book to solve their sleeping problem will easily understand the message has enabled me to better serve the reader.

The initial translation from Dutch to English was facilitated by www.GoTranscript.com, which yielded a text that gave us a good foundation to work with. Considerable edits were needed to adapt this level of translated English into colloquial language. Thank you again, Nora Smith, for this great and extensive job. If there even is such a thing as *just* an editing job, this certainly wasn't one of them. It required travel experience to have firsthand knowledge of cultural differences and to understand how to translate foreign experiences into locally relatable concepts. Since I had started the draft of this book on audio recordings, in Dutch, a lot of restructuring was needed as well as removing redundancy. For a big part of the way this book has shaped up, I am indebted to the skills of my editor.

Camara Cassin has helped to adjust and shift the content to be more emotionally engaging. Her viewpoints led to exciting discussions, which contributed to the birth of a smoother flow in our American English version and an overall great enhancement of the message.

Next to an extra editing round that yielded even more clarity and conciseness, Denise Kinsley suggested adding the summary sections at the end of the chapters. This section is particularly helpful for readers who want to actively work their way through the SoS Method and solve their sleeping problems.

This book has certainly been a team production. A big thanks to all of you!

Antoinetta Vogels,
Bellevue, WA, USA
HEALTHYSENSEOFSELF

ABOUT THE AUTHOR

Antoinetta Vogels is the founder of Healthy Sense of Self (United States) and author of the Sense of Self Method, a self-help program for people who want to get a good night's sleep no matter what!

Antoinetta was born in the Netherlands in 1946 and moved to Portugal when she was forty-five. A few years later, she settled down in the United States, where she still lives.

She has a teaching degree in French language and literature, and she studied music at the Royal Conservatory of Music in The Hague. For eighteen years she worked as a bassoonist in several well-established symphony orchestras. She is fluent in five languages and loves to travel. Ballroom dancing and music are a central part of her life.

Her insomnia began after the birth of her first child and lasted over twenty-five years. By studying her thoughts, feelings, and behavior, Antoinetta found that insomnia shows up when dependency on the approval of others thwarts the natural ability to sleep. The need to obtain optimal results to prove one's self-worth leads to the development of unhealthy patterns of motivation, which then lead to insomnia, anxiety, and depression.

Antoinetta's years of introspection and the resulting findings eventually guided her to the solution for her insomnia: restoring your sense of self is her recipe for permanently breaking free from chronic sleeping problems. She developed the Sense of Self Method to help others heal by teaching them the techniques she created to heal herself.

READ MORE FROM
ANTOINETTA VOGELS

Healthy Sense of Self: The Secret to Being Your Best Self!
(upcoming 3rd edition)

A Guided Journal to a Healthy Sense of Self: Thoughts to Inspire Peace Within and Around the World

The Sense of Self Method Workbook

The Sense of Self Method Online Course (available on https://www.Healthysenseofself.com)

Find us on Facebook and Instagram @HealthySenseofSelf

Healthy Sense of Self is also thriving in the Netherlands and in Italy:

www.Gezondzelfgevoel.nl
www.Sanosensodise.it

Printed in the United States
by Baker & Taylor Publisher Services